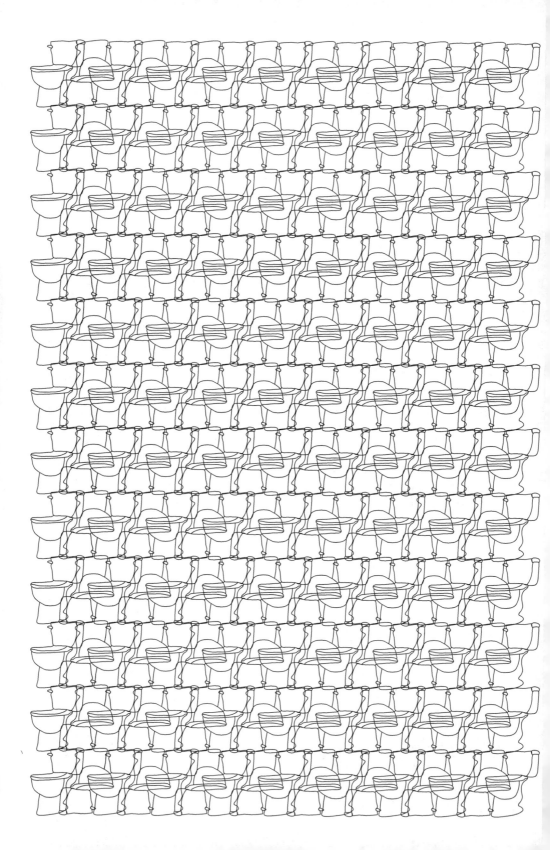

THE BODY DOESN'T KNOW HOW TO DIE

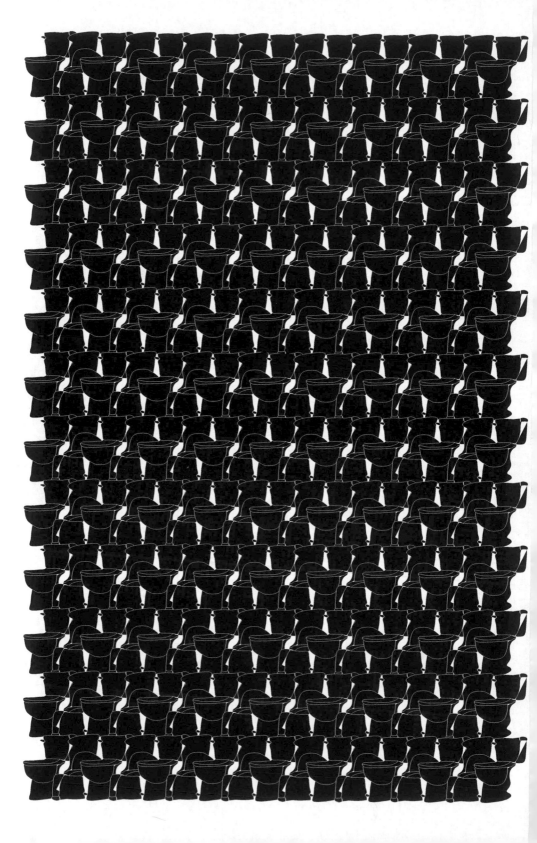

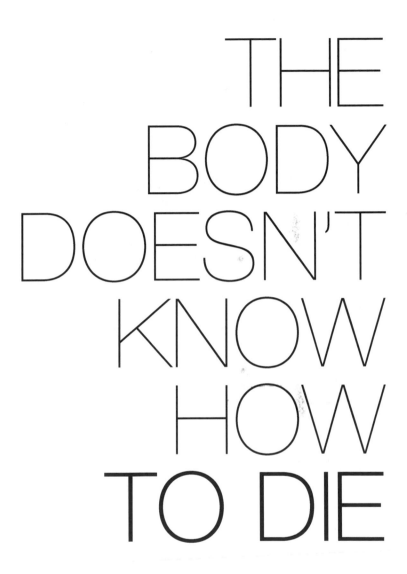

THE BODY DOESN'T KNOW HOW TO DIE

by

India Holloway

iUniverse, Inc.
Bloomington

The Body Doesn't Know How to Die:
The Body Only Knows How To Live, Heal, Mend and Rejuvinate

by India Holloway

India's Healthy Living/Life Well Institute
5835 W. Washington Blvd.
Culver City, CA 90230
Ph: 323-857-0800
Fx: 323-939-7951
E-mail: indiashealthyliving@gmail.com

Edited by Robin Quinn, Brainstorm Editorial
Book Design/Illustrations by Tasheka Arceneaux Sutton, Blackvoice Graphic Design Studio
Book Layout by James Arneson, JAAD Book Design

iUniverse books may be ordered through booksellers or by contacting:

iUniverse
1663 Liberty Drive
Bloomington, IN 47403
www.iuniverse.com
1-800-Authors (1-800-288-4677)

ISBN: 978-1-4697-7949-2 (sc)
ISBN: 978-1-4697-7951-5 (hc)
ISBN: 978-1-4697-7950-8 (e)

Library of Congress Control Number: 2012904727

Printed in the United States of America
iUniverse rev. date: 04/16/2012

Contents

*"If preventative measures and cleansing
were taught in medical schools,
many diseases we take for granted
would simply cease to exist."*

~ **Dr. Edward F. Group III, DC, ND, DACBN**

Foreword

by LAURA KOOBY

Director,
Education and Outreach,
Environmental Health Initiative,
American Association on Intellectual and
Developmental Disabilities

Every person has the right to live, work, play and pray in a safe and healthy environment. Research shows, however, that many environments are not fully protective of our health. In fact, our homes, work places, and outdoor spaces are quite often the very environments where we are exposed to chemicals that may be harmful to the human body.

Exposure to a wide range of potentially harmful chemicals from conception to death is unavoidable. There are about 80,000 registered chemicals in use in the United States. Approximately 3,000 chemicals are produced in quantities greater than 1 million pounds per year. Health effects are not always documented for these chemicals, and when they are, there is often weak regulation of these chemicals.

Some of the chemicals are neurotoxic, affecting the developing brain and the nervous system, and other chemicals are linked with diseases and disorders such as Cancer, learning disabilities, Autism, Asthma, Parkinson's Disease, Alzheimer's Disease, and even obesity.

It is well known that many factors can contribute to your personal health. This includes diet and exercise, genetic inheritance and lifestyle habits, and, significantly, your emotional and spiritual life. There are things we can do to stay healthy on a day-to-day basis: eat high-quality foods, drink clean water, breathe clean air free of cigarette smoke or other air contaminants like mold, and take care of the internal body.

Toxins can accumulate in the body in many places; your organs, fatty tissues, brain and bones are all susceptible to environmental exposures. Doing something protective of your health that safely removes toxic buildup can make tremendous improvements in overall health. One clear way to remove toxic buildup is through colonics, or the practice of flushing out the colon and small intestines in a gentle and safe way with the help of a professional.

The human body has an incredible ability to heal, and we can significantly impact our quality of life through taking simple steps toward health. The body wants to be healthy, and there are ways that you can support that through your daily habits.

It is important to support the body's natural ability to heal itself, especially if your personal genetic inheritance is fragile, your nutrition is not optimal, or when stress and lack of exercise threaten your quality of life. Keeping a healthy body in spite of these toxic exposures is an essential way to maintain a safe and healthy life.

The Poop Police

As a senior citizen, I wake up with virtually no aches or pains. I have great energy every day. I hit the ground running and continue until it's time to go to bed. I have no chronic diseases and take no medicine. Twenty-five years ago, I had little energy and more aches, pains, pings and pangs than a body has to right to have. In writing this book, my intention is help others feel as good as I do. My wish is for each of you to be free of destruction to the body. This is what we teach at Healthy Living Wholistic Health Care Services.

I am outraged when I hear of pharmaceutical companies that have been fined billions of dollars by the federal government for overstepping their bounds, i.e. bribing the medical doctors to continue dispensing prescriptions to enhance the big pockets and ignoring the fact that people are being harmed and dying from taking these drugs.

What's also disturbing is that the general public is not taught the real truth about their prescriptions – their dangers and the possible destruction to the body. Not enough is expressed as to why, with all the technology in the most advanced country in the world, **we are taught *disease care* rather than *health care*. Not how to manage your health instead of managing a disease.** And we are treated for diseases, rather than being told the truth about how the body can heal itself!

As a Colon Hydrotherapist, I think it is my duty to make you aware of just what Colon Hydrotherapy (CHT) is. Most people are not familiar with colonics (another term for CHT) will ask others who know just a little about it and get toilet loads of opinions and myths. Let me share the facts and dispel the myths.

Fact: No, CHT does not hurt. For newcomers, it can be a bit uncomfortable because, like with anything new, you do not know what to expect and may have a hard time relaxing. With an experienced therapist, a relaxation method can be instituted to assist. So just take a deep breath; you'll be fine.

Any harm the procedure could cause will be because the therapist is not versed enough or may not have had adequate training. For more info on finding a Board Certified Hydrotherapist, see www.i-act.org and Chapter 3, "Colon Hydrotherapy:

What you'll want to know … How it works." And if you can come to my offices in LA, you're welcome to make an appointment with me at Healthy Living located at the Life Well Institute (I have the highest level of CHT training).

DID YOU POOP TODAY?

Have you pooped today? Did you poop yesterday? Have you not pooped since last week? If you haven't pooped lately, something's wrong! Let's see now … if you eat three times a day and only poop every other day or every two days … and you only poop out tiny hard round pellets, that's a joke. Your poor body is on notice.

Do you wake up in the morning and have a hard time cranking it up (you keep hitting that snooze button)? Do you feel bloated and gassy following each meal, even if you eat just a little? Do you still feel bloated and gassy long after the meal is over? Then you're full of it! And if you're told this is normal, as bad as you feel, the person who told you that is full of it too!

FACT! It's time to empty that colon. One thing you can bank on if you have no energy is that you are full of toxic waste. Are you a little crazy these days? Are you mean, cantankerous and downright evil? Well, why shouldn't you be? The poop goes straight to your brain and will poison the grey matter.

Your body is talking to you and you're not listening! Somewhere down the line, you will suffer even more.

Making a good bowel movement, on the other hand, is like the angels singing. It's definitely a religious experience.

Over all else, my message to you is:

"MANAGE YOUR HEALTH – NOT A DISEASE!"

A Brief History of Colon Hydrotherapy

by INDIA HOLLOWAY

THERAPY OF THE COLON (large intestine) and its benefits have been known and practiced for many years. Dating back to ancient times, enemas were mentioned as early as 1500 BC in an Egyptian medical document called the "Eber Papyrus."

Hippocrates, Pare and Galen also advanced the use of enema therapy. In early times, people implemented enema treatments in a river by using a hollow reed to pour water into the rectum.

At an early time in America, enemas were a commonly used procedure to help maintain health and stave off disease. For example, before the departure of the Lewis and Clark expedition, a physician instructed them in the appropriateness of using enemas in cases of fever and illness. Our grandparents and great-grandparents grew up with the use of enemas as a widely accepted procedure for reversing the onset of illness.

In the early 1900s in Battle Creek, Michigan, John H. Kellogg, MD, extensively used colon therapy on some forty thousand of his patients. In 1917, he reported in **The Journal of the American Medical Association** that **in all but 20 cases** he used no surgery for the treatment of gastrointestinal disease in his patients.

The popularity of colon therapy reached its apex in the 1920s, 30s and 40s. At that time, colon irrigation machines were commonly seen, and regularly used as a standard practice in hospitals and doctor's offices. But in the ensuing 50 to 60 years, the public's use of, and access to, this valuable health treatment greatly decreased. The public's present lack of knowledge regarding this, and other personal healthcare treatments – together with the widely held belief by orthodox medicine that such treatments are no longer useful – may be the single most important factor in the current ill-health of our population.

> "In times past, knowledge of the bowel was more widespread and people were taught how to care for the bowel. Somehow, bowel wisdom got lost and it became something that no one wanted to talk about anymore."
>
> *–BERNARD JENSEN, D.C.*

Proper bowel management and health will never be achieved through the use of drugs and/or surgery. The answer can be found in a time-proven and natural approach ... Colon Hydrotherapy (CHT)!

COLON THERAPY – MAKING A COMEBACK!

Over the last 10 years, there has been a resurgence of interest in alternative medicine and personal healthcare responsibility. Once again, people are discovering the many health benefits of maintaining a strong and biologically sound colon. This return to using colon therapy has been bolstered by the development of sophisticated colon therapy techniques, which make these therapies both safe and convenient. I hope the grass-roots movement towards personal health responsibility, using alternative health therapies to restore and maintain superior health, will be joined by traditional healthcare practitioners.

According to the non-believers, no matter what research has been done on colonic irrigation and its benefits, the procedure is still deemed quackery. However, praise from those who have benefited from CHT far exceeds the complaints from the doubters.

I cannot think of a better way to jump-start the body's natural healing in today's society. Yet written information exposing positive references to the procedure over the last 50 to 100 years will never be good enough and certainly not credible for some, even if done by medical doctors and researched in the field of medicine. Why is that? What makes the many hundreds of thousands receiving colon irrigation and their experiences worthless in the eyes of the medical community? Perhaps it's because simple techniques are often pushed aside for ones that are more profitable for established medicine.

WE HAVE COME A LONG WAY, BABY!

DISCLAIMER

If you are ill or have been diagnosed with any disease,
please consult a medical doctor before attempting any natural healing program.
By using the information presented to you in this book,
you agree to take FULL responsibility for yourself.
It is important to always check with your medical practitioner.

Self-help requires intelligence, common sense,
and the ability to take responsibility for your own actions.
This information is provided with the hope that it may be helpful
for those who choose to take a greater responsibility for their own health.

If your health practitioner disagrees with your opinion,
find one who wants to listen to you! Your body will cure itself.
You have a right to cure yourself! It is certain that:

"A physician is a person that treats a patient until they die;
until their money is all gone; or until they are cured by nature."
~ DESCARTES

Qualified healthcare professionals are available just about everywhere! Find One!
If you suspect that you have a disease or health-related condition of any kind,
and you don't know what you should do, please learn and research ...
And learn from more than one source! Do your homework, and know your body very well.
Then follow your basic instincts.

If you are unable to learn, or if you are unable to help yourself,
you should contact a qualified healthcare professional
who practices natural and holistic therapy immediately.

Consult with your doctor before proceeding.

Again, this information is for people who are ready
to take full responsibility for their health.
If you are not one of those, then this information
is for informational purposes only.

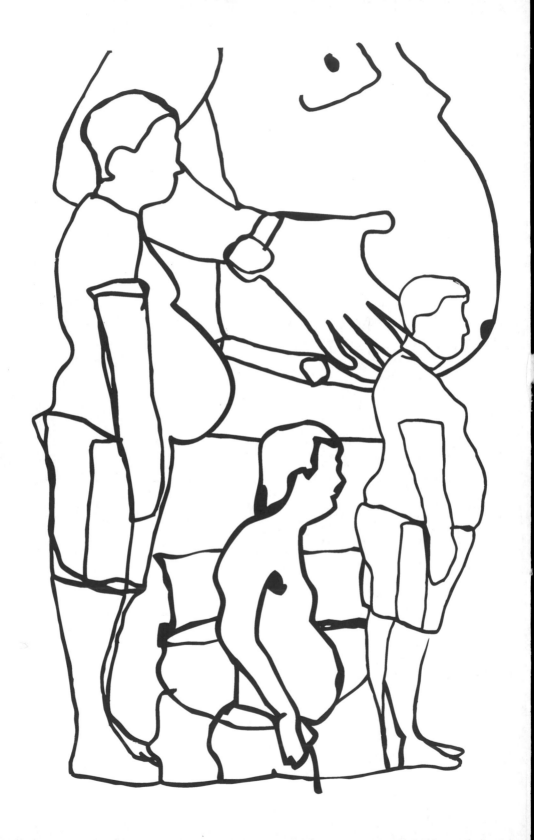

CHAPTER 1

Are You Listening To Your Body?

"GOOD GRIEF, why are my ankles always so swollen?" "Wholly crap! Why can't I lose weight?" "Why is there always a dull pain in my belly?" "Why am I so tired all the time?" "What causes this constant gas?" Blah blah blah …

You cannot win the battle of achieving your optimal weight or optimal health unless the body is balanced. What does that mean in the world of yo-yo diets, chemical imbalances, toxic foods and all that claims to be the cure for your particular health issue through the OCDs (over-the-counter drugs) and prescription medications? And the big one – having a "It's not gonna happen to me" attitude, which simply means "I do not wish to change"?

Everyones body is different, and your body may not conform to what seems to work for others when you're struggling with issues of mystery aches and pains. If it does work, it's only a temporary fix and you're back staring into the face of the same old demon once again – only this time you are a little older, other chemical changes have taken place, the body has possibly undergone undue stresses, etc., and you're more discouraged than ever. The fact is that many times you are still willing to dive head-first into the next, easy-appearing "Will this work for me?" diet, cure or remedy.

TRUTH: GOOD HEALTH IS A LIFESTYLE PROCESS.

CONSIDER THE FOLLOWING

Your body is an amazing instrument, and it is designed to not only keep you alive, but also to heal you when something goes wrong or breaks, tears, gets cut or is burned. You see it in one form or another on a daily basis. For instance, if you have a minor burn or if you cut your hand … *it heals!* The human body has a built-in genius that automatically heals on its own, given the proper time, conducive conditions, and, yes, *your assistance.*

The healing that takes place is not a miracle; it is really no big deal. The human body has a built-in DNA that only knows how to repair and get better. The one thing you have completely overlooked in this equation is that, as wonderful as the human body is, as magnificent a machine of automatic mechanism, it still needs *your help* to remain healthy.

Drugs are simply a patching up of your system. A drug manages your disease. A drug will not manage your health. Drugs are just a way to make you comfortable with your disease until you die. In other words, drugs give you *relief.* **It's easy to die.** It's not easy to live. It takes work and consistency in today's society. The reason that it is not so easy is that the whole of society has converted to dying the easy death with drugs and chemicals. To live the natural way requires investigation, research, management and a loyalty to one's body and the body's language.

Don't get me wrong … we should always honor our doctors and drugs for all the lives they save. You, however, are the most important factor in your own healthcare. Quite frankly, few doctors will tell you how to get healthy and stay healthy; how to reverse the effects of any disease. A doctor's job is to provide a diagnosis of a disease, treatment of a disease, or the cutting out of the disease. It isn't necessarily to tell you that you are doing something wrong, just that something specific *is* wrong. Do you really wish to take that medication "for the rest of your life," as you may be told?

YOUR BODY'S LANGUAGE

Your body has a language, and it speaks to you. Not to your doctor, your mom, your co-worker or the voodoo lady down the street. Everyone has an opinion, cure, solution or drug. Your body is speaking *to you,* and when you do not listen or will not listen, the consequences can be more than devastating. The consequences could be **fatal.**

This language comes to you in the form of *symptoms.* Pain is a symptom, a headache is a symptom. A blister on the toe is your body's way of possibly saying that those shoes are too damn tight and you've had them on too damn long, and the pinching and rubbing has caused your body to build up a defense. Hey! Get a half-size larger next time!

It is always advisable to check in with your doctor, especially when you have been ignoring your symptoms. The doctor's job is to look for clues by running tests to measure the state of your body. What is your blood pressure? What is your body's temperature? What are your cholesterol levels, your glucose (sugar) levels? And why the hell, when the doctor hits that knee with the little orange hammer, doesn't your foot kick him in the chin? (Ha ha!) Get a check-up so you know where to start. Ask questions.

But does your doctor believe you are a person and *not* just a symptom? Does s/he talk with you about prevention, show you measures you can do to reverse diseases and possibly get off the meds? Think about where you heard your first discussion on prevention and balance and how your body is capable of healing itself. It probably wasn't in your doctor's office.

Once you identify the problem, what needs to be done is to put your body in a position where it can heal itself. The human body is an extraordinary instrument, solidly capable of healing, mending, repairing and rejuvenating itself. You, however, must be that extraordinary human soul who will assist.

You are the main character in this equation. If you continue to pollute your body, don't keep it clean, are on self-destruct mode doing everything in your power to tear your body down and not help build it up … you are the enemy here.

LET'S TAKE THE ENEMY OUT OF THE PICTURE.

REMEMBER, IT'S EASY TO DIE! JUST GIVE UP! IT'S HARD TO LIVE; IT TAKES WORK … IT'S A JOB.

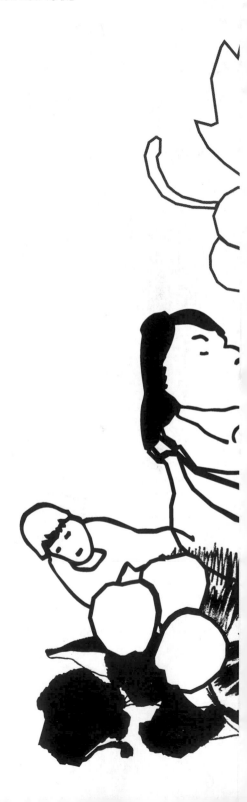

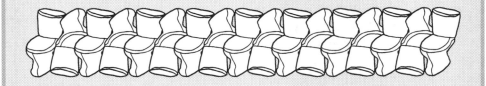

1. Drink plenty of water daily.

2. Eat organically grown foods. More importantly, eat the right combination of foods.

3. Get a good amount of rest. When the body sleeps, that's when it heals, mends and rejuvenates. Also, the body cannot digest foods and heal properly if you eat after 6 pm.

4. Keep stress at a minimum (stress alone can kill you).

5. Take your daily required supplements (do not skip them). Consistency is the key. I've had clients who tell me that they will not take supplements on the weekend just to give their body a rest. Does your heart stop for a rest?

6. Exercise routinely.

7. Keep the colon clean. The body cannot maintain its health or heal itself if it's full of toxic waste. Nutrients cannot be absorbed properly, and other major organs get jammed.

8. Your pH levels should always be balanced. It's a sign of good health.

9. Don't stuff yourself with food ... Eat until you are 80% full and stop! It takes your brain 20 minutes to catch up. I call it "the 80/20 Rule."

10. Eat six small meals daily (a meal could be an apple, an egg sandwich, a cup of tea, or peanut butter on a celery stick). Remember, you can't eat at 50 what you ate at 20.

Bonus tip: Watch out for sugar. It's a drug that will strip your body of its natural intelligence. Put your hands in the air – step away from that chocolate bar. Just step away.

More on all of this in the chapters ahead.

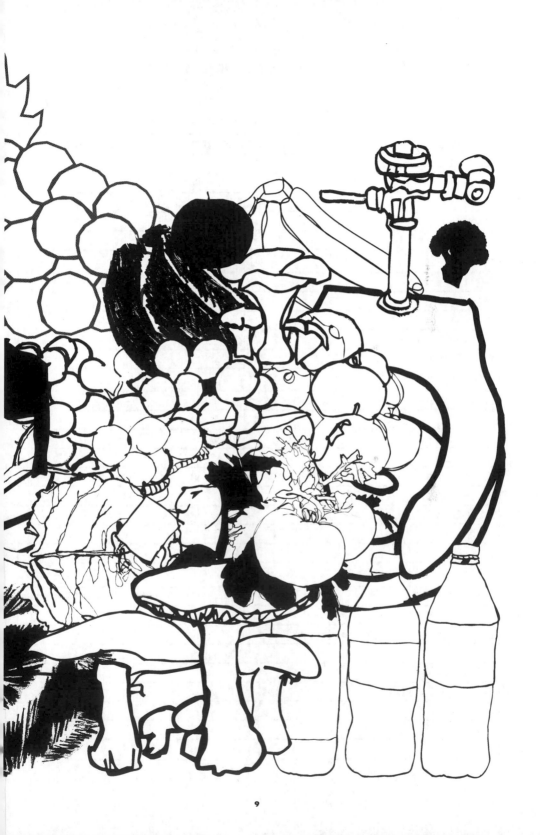

NEGATIVE HEALTH EFFECTS

According to the U.S. Government and product manufacturers,
the following is a partial list of chemical poisons found in products that are absorbed,
ingested or inhaled by the body before you even eat breakfast!
This list does not include the additional use of common household cleaners.

PRODUCT	KNOWN POISONOUS INGREDIENTS
MATTRESS & PILLOW	4 7
Air Freshner	1 4 7 8
Bath Soap*	3 4 5 6 7 8
Hair Shampoo	1 3 4
Hair Conditioner	1 4 8
Hair Spray	4 7
Skin Lotions	1 3 4 5 6 7
Shaving Cream	3 4
Aftershave Lotion	1 4 8
Skin Medication	1 3 4 5 6 7 8
Acne Medication	1 3 4 5 6 7 8
MOISTURIZERS	1 4 5 7 8
Antiperspirant	1 4 5 7 8
Cologne	1 4 7 8
Foot Deodorant	4 6 8
Toothpaste	3 4 5 6
Mouthwash	4 5 6 8
Plastic Glass	8
LAUNDRY	
Detergent*	1 3 4 5 6 7
Fabric Softener	3 4 5 7
Chlorine Bleach	1 2
Dry Cleaned Clothes	1 7
FEMININE PRODUCTS	
Lipstick, eye shadow, face powder, etc.	
Cosmetics	1 3 4 5 7 8
Facial Cleanser	3 4 8
Feminine Deodorant	4 7
Sanitary Napkins	4 7
Perfumes	1 4 7 8
Nail Polish	4 5 7 8

(*) Anti-bacterial products contain poisonous pesticides and fungicides as ingredients that create more serious health risks.

NEGATIVE HEALTH EFFECTS

1. Alcohols, Acid and Alkali: rashes, muscle weakness, headaches, dizziness, nerve damage, vision problems, sleeping problems, stomach cramps, disorientation, depression, coughing, respiratory problems, anemia, organ damage, fatigue, heart damage, cancer, death.

2. Chlorines: headaches, mental function difficulties, pulmonary edemas and heart disease, anemia, diabetes, gastrointestinal and urinary tract cancer, organ and gland cancer, severe eye problems, immune system breakdown, child development problems and more.

3. Detergents/Emulsifiers: strips skin of protective oils, skin irritation, scalp eruptions, interference with nutrient absorption, hair loss, allergic reaction, cataract formation, organ damage, reproductive damage, blindness, cancer.

4. Synthetic Fragrance & Dyes: allergic reactions, skin rashes, stomach upsets, muscular aches and pains, violent coughing and sneezing, irritability, vertigo, hyperactivity, convulsions, emotional and behavioral problems, Leukemia, Hodgkin's, emotional problems, ADD, multiple tumors, reproductive damage, headaches, dizziness, organ damage, depression, cancer.

5. Heavy Metals: abdominal cramps, nausea, joint and bone pain, muscle weakness, mouth sores, cancer, motor difficulties, reduced intelligence, brain disorders, short attention span, hyperactivity, emotional disorders, immune disorders, genetic damage, aging.

6. Pesticides & Fungicides: flu-like symptoms (fatigue, muscle and joint pain), stomach cramps, nervous system disorders, insomnia, memory loss, swelling of body parts, dizziness, genetic mutations, birth defects, gland tumors, organ damage, cancer, death.

7. Petrochemicals (chemicals derived from petroleum or natural gas): inhibits skin functions, pimples, rashes, splitting nails, sensitivity to sun, headaches, premature aging, allergic reactions, depression, fatigue, intestinal gas, asthma, respiratory failure, immune system disorders.

8. Preservatives (synthetic): headaches, skin rashes, eye damage, asthma, respiratory problems, tumors, cancer, digestive problems, mental confusion, organ damage, muscle weakness and cramps, loss of motor control, joint pain, reproductive damage, etc.

When using common household cleaners in the shower, on mirrors, toilet, etc., you inhale and absorb a whole new range of poisonous chemicals that can damage the organs, eyes, central nervous system and respiratory system.

Day after day, week after week, year after year, people may be unaware that they are being exposed to numerous poisonous chemicals found in common, everyday household and personal care products. By themselves, there is reason for concern; but when you combine them in your body, there is reason to worry.

If a product has a warning on the label, it is poison! What is the cumulative effect on our health after using many, many products that contain small amounts of dangerous poisonous chemicals?

We spend every night breathing vapors from chemical poisons in the mattress or pillow and sleeping between sheets washed in poison. A typical US family might start the day grooming with a shower/bath (soap, shampoo, hair conditioner), brush teeth, shave, as well as using colognes, perfumes, hairsprays, etc., in an enclosed area. We are using many products containing poisonous ingredients. Then we all dress with clothes washed in poison.

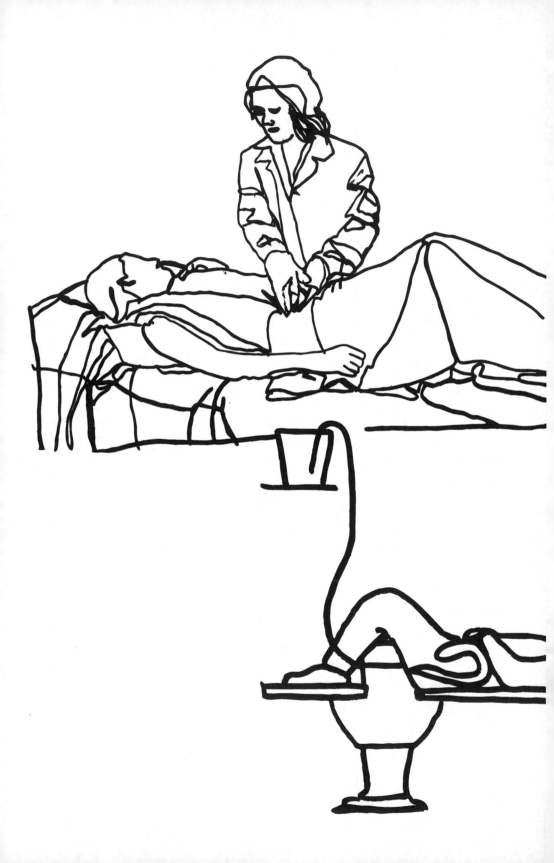

CHAPTER 2

Why Clean The Colon?

CHILDREN INTUITIVELY LEARN by imagination, and by rote, a mechanical process of learning: *they learn what they live.* You may not remember when you were being potty-trained – you can best believe it was not from a pocket manual. Children aren't hung up on words and instructions or interpretations of completed printed symbols. In other words, for children, learning is doing and thinking, like singing the ABC song to learn the alphabet. There are those who read every book they can find on health and health issues but do increasingly less about their well-being. Thus they remain unhealthy by being unmotivated about doing the right things. The body does not automatically heal because you've read the sacred words. Now let's go back to basics.

**USE YOUR GOOD COMMON SENSE,
USE YOUR IMAGINATION AND FOLLOW YOUR INTUITION.**

Death begins in the colon. Don't believe it? Ask any coroner.
Autopsies often reveal colons that are plugged up to 80 percent with waste material."
- VEGETARIAN TIMES, MARCH, 1998

WHY CLEAN THE COLON?

There are several major reasons I've identified through study, research and years of observation why, if that colon is nasty, you may grow old feeding your diseases or die young giving diseases their fill. Of all the polite topics of conversation, the state of one's intestines is probably at the bottom of most people's lists. Let's face it: Irritable bowel syndrome, constipation, gas, diverticulitis and colon cancer are simply not things we like to discuss.

CONSTIPATION

A constipated system is one in which transit time (the time it takes for food to move through your system from when you eat until you poop it out) is slow and the consistency of the stool can cause strain (which over time may lead to hemorrhoids, varicose veins, or other mechanically induced problems). The longer the "transit time," the longer the toxic waste matter sits in the bowel, which allows proteins to putrefy (rot), fats to go rancid (spoil), and carbohydrates to ferment. This all spells out toxins and smells out G-A-S!

A good cleansing program should always begin by removing the waste in your colon, followed by kidney and liver cleanses in that order. It is a fact that if you attempt to clean your liver, blood or lymph system without first addressing a waste-filled bowel (the colon), the excreted toxins will only get recycled back into your body.

This is what you don't want to know: If you have an inherent weakness in your body, check out your family's health history and chances are you have inherited those weak genes. You are giving those nasty genes food to surface by! Eighty to ninety percent of all diseases are fueled by your diet.

It has been proven that much more effective and long-term results of good health have been realized by people who have cleansed their colon first. The body can heal itself and detoxify more efficiently if the colon is cleansed, rather than when the colon is full of toxic waste. **DON'T FEED THOSE NASTY GENES!**

Meat has no fiber, "ham"-burger has no fiber, pizza has very little fiber, and dairy is constipating – especially cheese. What are your children eating? What are you eating? Show me a constipated kid and I'll show you a parent who's not making regular bowel movements and/or has a bloated, distended belly.

"Most people, including many physicians, do not realize that 80 percent of your immune system is located in your digestive system, making a healthy gut a major focal point if you want to maintain optimal health. Remember, a robust immune system is your number one defense system against ALL disease."

–DR. JOSEPH MERCOLA

FROM ARTICLES.MERCOLA.COM

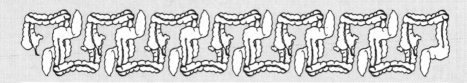

TIP FOR AVOIDING OR GETTING RID OF CONSTIPATION

Hydrate: Drink plenty of water or herbal teas. (Drink half of your weight in ounces of water per day.) The most important time to hydrate is first thing in the morning. You should drink 20-30 ounces of water with a pinch of sea salt (see Chapter 9, "Blood, Sweat & Tears") straight down upon awaking ... before your feet hit the floor. Drink two more 6-8 ounce glasses of water before noon, the last glass or bottle of 8 ounces just before going to bed. Consume the rest throughout the day. A good gauge is 4 ounces every half hour.

Of course, the proper amount of water you should drink depends upon a number of factors, including your gender, age, level of activity, and environment.

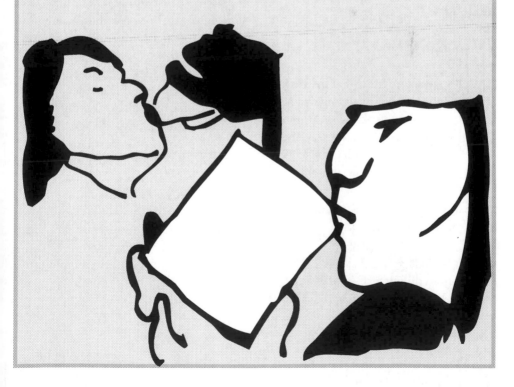

One of the most frequent bowel problems that people experience today is constipation. Constipation is closely associated with diabetes, and it's the number one problem among children (that is outrageous!). Constipation is generally attributed to a low-fiber diet and a lack of sufficient water (dehydration) and – for goodness sake – eating too much fast food, sugary food and not chewing your foods sufficiently (a product of our fast-paced society). All of this causes our poop to become condensed, compressed and sticky. What does it spell? **C-O-N-S-T-I-P-A-T-I-O-N.**

WHAT IS IT ABOUT THE COLON THAT CAN MAKE IT APPEAR SO WEAK VULNERABLE AND HELPLESS?

Most live to eat, not eat to live. YOU KNOW WHAT I'M TALKING ABOUT.

1. It is important to know that there are more and more individuals born with some sort of colon weaknesses. From the time this person is born, there have been issues of slow elimination from a sluggish colon. I see them now as adults, and it has progressed into yet a larger issue.

2. Eat less sugary and carbohydrate foods (pizza is rat food).

3. Check the side-effects of any medication. FYI. Medications that can cause constipation: dihydrocodeine, diuretics and those containing aluminum, calcium and iron. And for sure, the muscle relaxers. The colon is made of muscle tissue and you want to relax it? I'm just saying!

4. Exercise. Since the colon is muscle tissue, it needs exercise.

5. Go to your children's school and check the restrooms (would you go there?).

6. Chew your foods well (approximately 15 to 20 times before swallowing).

When constipated, there is an infrequent urge to poop; however, the stool is hard and difficult to pass. Whenever you strain to poop, you risk fissures (tears) and/or hemorrhoids. When you go for too long without getting that toxic waste out of the colon, the abdomen may become distended and crampy; and more often than not, disturbing bowel sounds and major stinky gas occur. All can result in a somewhat embarrassing experience if not put in check.

Ask your doctor or other healthcare professional if s/he can recommend a good cleansing program. (A stool softener will not do the trick.) If you've been dining on the Standard American Diet (SAD), stool softeners are a joke and the OTC (over-the-counter) laxatives are damaging, dehydrating and can be too harsh. Herbal laxatives are a better alternative.

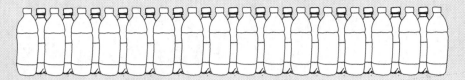

WATER

SYMTOMS OF DEHYDRATION

Every function the body performs requires water. Water is essential for your body to function properly. It flushes toxins out of your organs, carries nutrients throughout the body, and provides a moist environment for sensitive tissues and organs like those arthritic fingers and knees. The body will begin to send signals to your brain when it is not properly hydrated; it will produce the following symptoms:

1. HEADACHE (And you take a pain pill and drink a soda.)

2. THIRST (And you drink juice, soda and beer.)

3. DRY MOUTH (And you suck on a mint.)

4. MUSCLE WEAKNESS (And you lie down and sleep.)

5. FATIGUE OR LETHARGY (And you reach for a cup of coffee, a soda or a candy bar.)

6. DIZZINESS (And you pick up the phone to make a doctor's appointment.)

7. LIGHTHEADEDNESS (Water carries oxygen to the brain.)

Despite the fact that thirst is always a good indication of the need for water, you should not wait until you are thirsty to drink. And if you do, DON'T DRINK SODA.

LET'S EXPLORE SOME OF THE EFFECTS OF WATER DEFICIENCY

1. Low blood pressure
2. Clotting of blood
3. Kidney malfunction
4. Severe constipation

HOW ABOUT SOME OF THE FUNCTIONS OF WATER IN THE HUMAN BODY?

1. Water is essential for digesting food. It is also important for getting rid of various toxic elements from the body, in the form of urine, sweat and fecal matter. Approximately 70-80% of your poop is water.

2. Water helps to cushion our joints and prevents shock to these areas of our body.

3. Water present in blood is the carrier of oxygen and nutrients to all our body cells.

4. Water present in lymph (a fluid that is part of our immune system) helps the body to fight against various diseases.

5. Water helps to regulate and maintain our body temperature. Think about those secret summers, ladies. (Men, that refers to women's hot flashes.)

6. Water prevents dehydration, and thus it helps to maintain proper metabolism in our body.

me
ea
no fi

t has
ber....

The bottom line is that constipation is a result of the muscular action of the colon that is not functioning properly, and the main culprit is what you've been eating all these years or what you recently had to eat too much of. Next in line is stress and time-restraint. And for those who find it difficult to poop anywhere other than home ... my advice is: *get over it!*

I have found over the years that there are certain professions in which the problem of constipation has popped up consistently: Nurses, school teachers, flight attendants, female police officers and hair stylists. Percentage-wise, they make up the bulk of my clientele. (This truly should be considered covered by workers compensation.)

THE COLON AND ITS CONNECTION TO CANCER

The longer your intestine is exposed to putrefying, rotting and fermenting food, the greater your risk of developing disease. Yes, even cancer. Even while making one bowel movement a day, you will still have at least two meals worth of waste matter putrefying in your colon at all times. Your body is not made to hold onto waste. This extra waste is what leads to disease.

A perfect world would be void of junk food, pollutants, human-made toxins in the foods we eat, clothes we wear, water we drink; plus, the chemicals we put on and into our bodies. After all, our skin is transdermal; if we put stuff in our hair or on our skin, we might as well drink it. Think about that now! Birth control patches and no smoking patches? Tell me this; where do the chemicals go when the patch is finished doing its job? Does it osmos itself? Or does it collect into fat cells, dump into the colon perhaps?

I'm telling you we ask a lot of our colon and it needs your help.

Talk with anyone you know who has been diagnosed with colorectal (colon/ rectum) cancer. Ask them how often they eliminate (poop) and you will get varying answers. You could poop practically every day, two to three times a day, and still end up with colorectal cancer. Why? According to research, one common factor is what you feed your body. Now think about this.

When you show symptoms of colon disease, you are already in a crisis. That being said, you could have symptoms as seemingly benign as hiccups or as traumatic as severe abdominal pain and violent vomiting, which would show the early signs of a disease. It's time to clean house. If a body's been diagnosed with cancer, it didn't just jump in out of the blue. It started 5, 10, maybe even 20 years ago. And in the African-American community, colorectal cancer (CRC) is diagnosed in one out of every two persons.

Let's put it all together. Faulty living habits and faulty elimination will cause at least 90% of the toxic buildup and poisons in the body. This will no doubt put your body in a position where it cannot heal itself.

When you consider colorectal, prostate and breast cancers as cancers that are

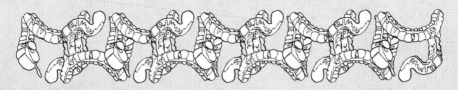

SYMPTOMS

Symptoms are your body's way of saying, "FIX IT!"

1. HEADACHE (And it's not your typical hangover.)

2. ACID INDIGESTION (And you haven't eaten in five hours.)

3. LOW BACK PAINS (Out of nowhere)

4. SLUGGISHNESS (And you've just slept eight hours.)

5. DRYNESS AND STIFFNESS (And you're only 23 years old.)

6. SYMPTOMS YOUR DOCTOR CANNOT EXPLAIN (And they've performed every reasonable test.)

These symptoms could come from almost anywhere and be from almost anything. However, a lifestyle change and good colon cleanse are definitely in order!

REASONS FOR COLORECTAL CANCER IN BLACK AMERICANS ARE

1. LACK OF PREVENTION. More often than not, trying to get the average black male to the doctor for normal check-ups is like pulling teeth from a live crocodile. Unlikely, unless symptoms are occurring, such as pain and/or bleeding. You are now in a crisis, my friend; prepare for takeoff. Chances are that you are already three to five years too late.

2. POOR DIET. More than half of all African-American women are obese or overweight. And according to the American Cancer Society, colorectal cancer in women is higher than in men.

Note: Symptoms of colon cancer include unusual change in bowel habits, change in stool, signs of bleeding, fatigue, weight loss, and feeling that the bowel does not empty completely. Get to know your body, and take care of it! Don't let this disease happen to you!

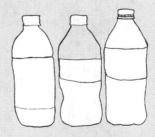

"ham
burg
has
fibe

True Story

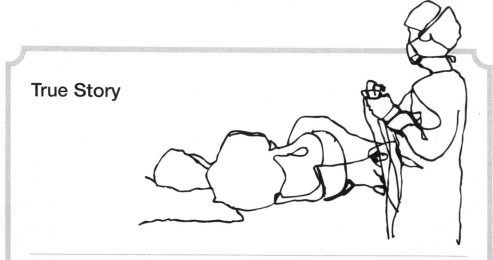

One of the benefits of cleaning the colon is that common joint-pain subsides.

I have a client, a nurse, who did not concede to colon hydrotherapy. However, during an annual physical check, she was advised that a colonoscopy was necessary as a routine screening for cancer. The procedure would look at changes in the lining of the colon known as inflammatory disorders.

Prior to her procedure, she took major medications for years for joint pain, primarily pain in the knees. Side note: the anti-inflammatory medications for arthritis are extremely difficult on the liver and kidneys and one of the side effects is constipation.

For those of you who have never had a colonoscopy, you are expected to clean the rectum and colon, which must be completely emptied of stool for the procedure to be performed. In general, the preparation consists of consumption of a special cleansing solution (a product named "HalfLytely" – which contains polyethylene glycol [Peg] 3350, sodium chloride, sodium bicarbonate, and potassium chloride – along with bisacodyl delayed release tablets) PURCHASED AT YOUR LOCAL PHARMACY (nick-named "Rocket Fuel"), or several days of clear liquids, laxatives and enemas prior to this procedure.

She had her colonoscopy and at the same time noticed the pain in her knees were completely gone. In fact, she felt WONDERFUL! Her colon was completely cleaned and she was off the inflammatory meds for one whole month.

A year or so later, she heard talk of colonics and decided to try it based on her clinical experience with the colonoscopy Rocket Fuel. Needless to say, I've got a new believer.

90% curable when caught in time, you would think a check-up over death would be the most obvious choice.

**HERE ARE SOME
SOBERING THOUGHTS**

Fear will keep you from a check-up and from knowing the truth. A diagnosis gives you either the excuse to give up and die or a chance to live a long, productive life. Your system can become continuously self-polluting from all the "poisonous gases" that are caused by the foods your body can only tolerate for so long. You know well which foods your body hates (all you lactose-intolerant ice-cream eaters, gas-passing regulars); these toxins can enter your bloodstream, irritating your organs and joints and causing you even more grief.

Try not eating foods that cause you physical discomfort and unsettling reactions. Not knowing gives you the excuse to continue doing all the wrong things (i.e. not exercising, eating crazy, and taking those insane medical OTC medications that just disguise or cover up the symptoms) or you just ignore the problem altogether.

Alternating between constipation and diarrhea, or having diarrhea alone also indicates that there is foul matter in your intestines.

Please do not think it's funny when dad cracks a good fart that makes the dog run barking or your kid screams out for "MOM!" That constant foul smell is an indication of something brewing in there. Get it checked out.

Finally, the serious problems of cancer and various immune system dysfunctions begin with a toxic bowel, so let's clean house. The only temple you will own until you die just may be the nastiest thing you know.

The long-held belief of some health professionals is that many people just have fewer bowel movements than others. This is true, but they also neglected to share that those having fewer bowel movements are harboring a fertile breeding ground for serious diseases and possibly death. Infrequent or poor quality bowel movements over an extended period of time are very hazardous to your health as well. Mold grows in deep dark moist places.

Have you ever wondered why, when you cannot poop, you may develop a headache? Wondered why you have a coated tongue? Did you think foul breath was just from bad gums or rotted teeth? Indeed that rough skin could look better. You may also find yourself out of sorts, not up to par and downright evil. Well, your body is yelling for help! Your body has seven channels of elimination. It's time to cleanse.

All we have to do is to truly understand that the single greatest confrontation our body faces is the effective removal of wastes and toxins from the colon; or from the body, period. Everything coming out of your body is waste – blood, sweat and tears! It's all waste – mucus, ear wax, etc. You breathe in oxygen, you breathe out … guess what? Carbon dioxide, waste! What goes in will find a way out – sometimes that is good to you. Other times … well, there is disease.

pizza
has
fiber

a
zero
...

Pooping, more formally referred to as bowel movements, should be accomplished **a minimum of two to three times a day, or a bare minimum of once a day.** And when you poop, your stool should be at least one inch in diameter and approximately a foot to a foot and a half long. Less than that means you're holding onto waste for future damage. Call it what you want… then call me "Damage Control"! As a colon hydrotherapist, my job is to move waste.

TRANSIT TIME

As noted earlier, the longer the transit time, the longer the toxic waste matter sits in the bowels, allowing proteins to putrefy, fats to become rancid, and carbohydrates to ferment. The longer the body is exposed to rotting food in the intestines, the greater the risk of developing disease.

Gastroenterologist Dr. Anthony Bassler tells his colleagues: "Every physician should realize that the intestinal toxemias (poisons) are the most important primary and contributing causes of many disorders and the diseases of the human body."

AUTOINTOXICATION

V.E. Irons, a well-known herbalist, says, "There's only one disease among humans and that's autointoxication, and everything else is a symptom of that."

Retained debris in the colon leads to the absorption or re-absorption of toxins, resulting in systemic intoxication (autointoxication or self-poisoning of the body). You cannot live like that. Colon hydrotherapy (colonics) or colon irrigation is a sure way to re-educate the colon, detoxify and hydrate the body, and eliminate putrefied matter to avoid autointoxication. The major common factor of this problem is found in the digestive tract.

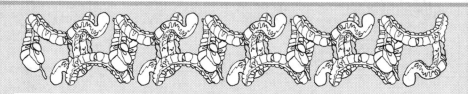

KNOWLEDGE IS POWER

If your pain or symptoms are so severe that you go to the doctor or are rushed to a hospital out of fear and lack of knowledge … this could be your death sentence.

But if you instead approach the health of your body with knowledge, you have strength. You should know your body well enough to ask the appropriate questions and even know the general answers or what is not appropriate for you. That is power and knowledge, and it makes it hard to accept the wrong information.

True Story

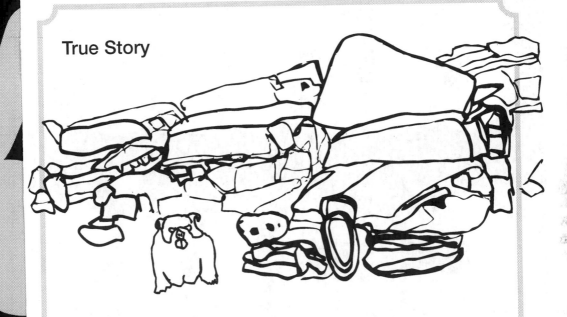

My husband was hospitalized for two months for knee-replacement surgery. He had been scheduled to be released one week following the surgery. Two weeks following the operation, he had not had a bowel movement and he was still in the hospital. They fed him three times a day and noted when he did not eat. No notes were taken when he did not poop. As a colon hydrotherapist, I was crazed and beside myself running around, pulling my hair out, trying to figure out how to pump poop out of this man who had major pain, tubes stuck everywhere (except up his butt), and whose disposition was that of a junkyard dog. He would not take my suggested herbs due to his concern that they might interfere with his prescribed meds. So I was forbidden to enter the junkyard. When this bloated misery was more miserable due to the constipation than the surgery itself, I received the request, "Make me poop!" I was on it. With simple remedies and major prayers, I finally got the poop to flow and, let me tell you, the colon was so warped from the meds. His stools were jet black and the consistency of jelly mud.

Imagine the relief and the shock. "What was that? If it moved, I'd swear it was a baby." Did I see it? Oh, and yes, I even saw a smile from the junkyard dog.

Healing is much more rapid when the body is free of toxins.

From major halitosis (bad breath), to chronic fatigue, to a lack of vitality and headaches, how many of your family members, friends and colleagues do you know who are sailing on this ship? Well, guess what! The boat's about to sink.

It's not if. But *when will it go down?*

When you don't make a poop but once every three or four days, those headaches escalate and subside only when you can finally let loose. As noted, two to three bowel movements per day is actually what a healthy person should be having. For each meal we eat, we should poop something out. Quoting the experts, the Royal Society of Medicine of Great Britain has stated, "More than sixty-five different health challenges are caused by a toxic colon."

How about when you're feeling so bad, tired and fatigued, listless, bloating and gassy that you go to your doctor. S/he gives you a stool softener or suggests that you drink the pink liquid chalk and says, "See me in 30 days."

Most doctors ignore this silent damage that becomes the silent killer that slowly creeps in and takes over the body. In more cases than not, the problem is not addressed until you are in a crisis.

Stop and think for a moment. You have five eliminatory organs and a total of seven systems of elimination – all made to get rid of waste. Your eliminatory organs are your lungs, kidneys, skin, colon and liver – all made to dump toxins. You are a sewer (it comes in; it goes out); you are not a cesspool. You are made to rid your body of waste, not store it.

FOR EVERY YEAR YOU HAVE CAUSED YOUR BODY DISTRESS AND DIS-EASE, IT WILL TAKE A MONTH TO REPAIR ... YOU DO THE MATH.

BE PROUD OF YOUR POOP. REMEMBER, "A DAY WITHOUT POOPING IS LIKE A DAY WITHOUT SUNSHINE."

You could cleanse other parts of the body, such as the liver, lungs and kidneys, and not cleanse the colon. However, the effectiveness of the detox will not be there.

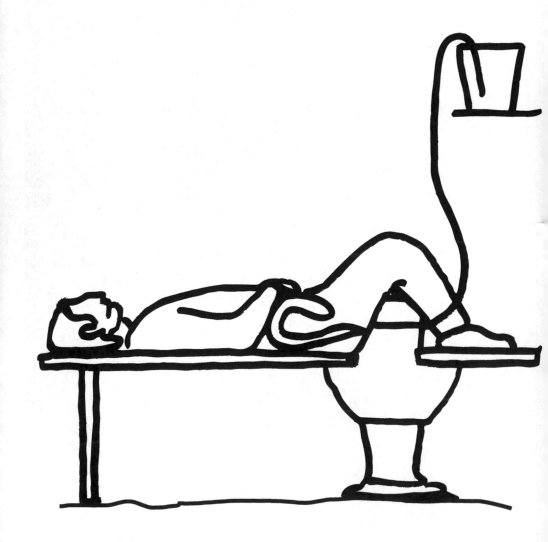

CHAPTER 3

Colon Hydrotherapy: What You'll Want to Know... How it Works

ALSO KNOWN AS "colonics," colon hydrotherapy (CHT) is a gentle irrigation/cleansing process designed to eliminate toxic waste from the large intestine. It is a technical skill performed by a trained and certified colon therapist. The procedure is performed using a FDA-recognized colonic device. The fluid or liquid that comes from the equipment is filtered water – no soap, saline or chemicals are involved.

The filtered water is used to flush the entire colon, removing the buildup from around the colon walls. You should not expect the debris to be removed in one visit; it may take several colonics to accomplish this.

WHAT ARE THE BENEFITS OF COLON HYDROTHERAPY?

Dr. Bernard Jensen, a world-renowned chiropractor/nutritionist, taught that disease, as well as health, begins in the colon. If you're interested in improving or maintaining your health, having a strong functioning colon will be essential. Together with the liver, kidneys, lungs and skin, your colon is responsible for eliminating old waste from the body. However, over time, your colon may lose its ability to properly eliminate all waste from the gastrointestinal tract due to a combination of poor diet, improper food-combining, drug intake, unhealthy lifestyle and/or stress. You may be aware that many drugs (recreational and prescription) cause constipation.

When it is compromised, the colon may become saturated with harmful toxins. And through "autointoxication" (which you learned about in the last chapter), these toxic substances can be transported into the bloodstream to the point that the lymphatic and circulatory systems, as well as the lungs and kidneys, become overburdened and expose you to serious health risks.

Colon hydrotherapy supports the restoration of good health by:

- Clearing the colon of old, hardened waste-material and harmful toxins
- Helping to re-establish proper pH balance to the body
- Assisting in stimulating the immune system
- Allowing freer passage of nutrients into the blood stream
- Working to prevent the absorption of toxins by fostering a healthy mucosa (along the lining of the colon)
- Providing a favorable environment for the bacteria and microflora that support digestion
- Strengthening peristaltic (natural muscular contraction) activity in the colon, and thereby toning the large intestine
- Promoting a return of normal, regular bowel movements
- Hydrating of the body from the water that flows through the colon
- Rejuvenating the entire system, the same as a good hot bath or shower. It's like a day at the spa; it's like a singing opera.

A healthy colon is vital to living a life free of degenerative disease! When putting together a health program, remember that colon hydrotherapy can be beneficial. Make it a part of your plan.

FREQUENTLY ASKED QUESTIONS

Is colon hydrotherapy similar to an enema?

The two processes are somewhat similar. However, an enema only deals with about 6 to 12 inches of the colon, while colon hydrotherapy is designed to flush the entire 5 to 5-1/2 feet of the large intestine.

How does CHT work or how is it performed?

(Note: The answer below describes the "Closed System" of Colon Hydrotherapy. You'll find further info on the Closed System and a description of the Open System later in this chapter.)

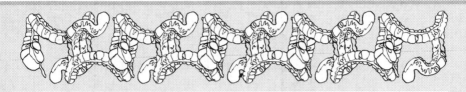

CONSIDER THESE STATISTICS

According to the Consumer Healthcare Products Association, annual over-the-counter sales for laxatives were $822 million in 2009 – up from $708 million in 2006. Seems like folks are getting clogged up more than ever!

Sales in 2009 for OTC heartburn remedies (including anti-gas) were $1,277 million.

The Center for Disease Control reports that close to 140,000 people were diagnosed with colorectal (colon/rectum) cancer in 2006. Their stats also show that 26,801 men and 26,395 women died that year from colorectal cancer.

These numbers are crazy, as this is the most preventable form of cancer that threatens Americans.

Digestive system cancers (including colon cancer) were estimated to be the second deadliest type of cancer in the US in 2010, following genital system cancers.

REMEMBER, HEALTH BEGINS IN THE COLON!

While you lie on the table, the colon hydrotherapist infuses water into the colon through the rectum. Depending on the amount of buildup in the colon, anywhere from 2 cups to 2 gallons of water will be used.

Over a period of 35 to 45 minutes, filtered water gently flows in and out of the colon dragging out old fecal matter. There is no need to leave the table to expel the water. The passage of the water, in and out of the colon, is controlled by the therapist who operates the device.

Does it hurt?

Absolutely not. There should be NO pain. However, if you work with someone who is not proficient in their skills, you may have a bad experience. With a skilled professional, you should be no more than just a little uncomfortable. The speculum can feel like a turd stuck half in and half out. However this sensation dissipates after about 5 minutes as your focus is redirected to other things, such as sensations in the feet, knees and/or legs. There might be some slight cramping in the lower left side of belly, etc. All sensations are fleeting and mild in nature; most people do not witness them at all.

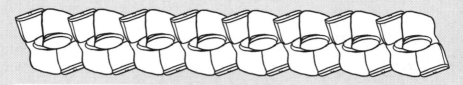

Colon Preparation Instructions

It's important that you stick to the following preparations to assure a successful CHT session.

If the client does not eliminate at least once a day, I recommend that they take (to begin) 2 Herbal Capsules (i.e. Dr. Schulze Intestinal Formula #1) at bedtime with a full glass of water (alkaline water or spring water with lemon) for two to three days before their appointment. These Herbal Capsules are available through my website.

1. Eat light the day before and the day of the colonic (no big steak dinner the night before!). You might have a salad with shrimp for dinner the previous night. Have a light breakfast that day – such as fruit and/or oatmeal. Have a salad for lunch. Eat fruit in the afternoon.

2. Eat no bread the day of the colonic, or pizza.

3. Eat nothing that's salty that day. Salt makes the body retain water. Eat no chips or popcorn. Most soups are too salty.

4. Drink no coffee that day. Have tea in the morning. Coffee is an acid and a stimulant. The tea will assist you in weaning off of the coffee.

5. Have no sweets or sugar (or cut way down) for three days before your appointment.

6. Also avoid these foods for three to five days before your appointment:

   - Bananas
   - Chocolate
   - Carob
   - White flour
   - Candy
   - Potatoes
   - Fried foods
   - Cheese
   - Pickles

7. CONSUME NO FOOD FOR 1 HOUR BEFORE THE COLON HYDRO-THERAPY SESSION. Your belly should be mostly empty when you get to the appointment.

8. In addition, incorporate my general recommendations for healthy eating on a daily basis (for more information, see Chapter 8 "It's Not a Diet; It's a Lifestyle Change"):

   a. NO red meat

   b. NO white bread

   c. Drink water each day, half your-body weight in ounces.

So if you weigh 140 pounds, you would drink at least 70 ounces of water a day. Drink 20 of these ounces first thing in the morning*, and two more 8-ounce glasses of water before noon. Drink your last 8-ounce glass of water at bedtime. Drink your remaining ounces in the afternoon and evening. Be sure to drink alkaline water or add freshly squeezed lemon juice to each glass. (Lemon helps quicken the removal of waste or unwanted toxins from the body.) *For those who can drink more: Drink up to 30 ounces upon rising in the AM.

Attention menstruating women! It is not unusual and quite natural for your menstrual cycle to come on prematurely when you begin to detox. Most colon hydrotherapists will still want you to keep your appointment. Call ahead to confirm.

Can I lose weight with CHT?

Yes, but colon hydrotherapy is not a weight-loss program. The weight you lose is waste, poop, sewage; and I've extracted as much as 10 pounds of the stuff in one visit. The average individual will leave behind, as a token of appreciation, 1 to 5 pounds each visit. All in all, it is a great jumpstart to any weight loss program.

How often should I get a colonic?

How often one should have colonics depends on the diet, stress level, health, age, and how successful a colonic is at moving the impacted waste matter. It is advised to have a colonic until mucus is no loner visible in the release water. The general recommendation, depending on the individual, may be an initial series of three, five, or sometimes eight to ten sessions being completed before going on a maintenance program (usually monthly, quarterly or bi-annually).

Who can get CHT? ... The sick? The healthy? The good, the bad, the ugly?

One thing is certain, when you speak with a qualified colon hydrotherapist, that individual should ask you questions to be sure there are no contraindications (health conditions that say you should not do this). If there are none, you qualify ... go for it.

AFTER THE COLONIC

Following your colonic:

1. You may feel sluggish for two or three days.
2. You may experience symptoms of a cold.
3. You may witness a skin rash or breakout.
4. You may not have a bowel movement for two or three days.
5. You may feel slight swelling of your lymph areas (for example, under the arms or in the groin area).
6. If you've had a previous history of constipation, you may experience a slight headache.

Not to worry ... these are common occurrences after receiving a colonic. The poisons and toxins in your body have been stirred up and are on the move. The toxins find exits any way they can when the colon is purged. It is unnatural for your body to hold on to years of putrefied waste and toxins.

After the colonic, one can feel more peaceful, lighter, cleaner and more energized. On rare occasions, if there has been a long-standing condition of constipation or continuous health problems, a slight headache or fatigue may be experienced after the first or second colonic session. If this is so, a short rest will help restore one's equilibrium. Also, drink plenty of water. You might take a detox bath too (see Chapter 7 for bath instructions).

Because the colon has been cleared of solid matter, it may take one or two days before it fills up again and normal bowel movements are resumed. Some water is absorbed through the colon wall during a colonic, and one may notice an increased need to urinate for a few hours afterwards. The beneficial effects of this flushing of the kidneys may be enhanced by drinking a few glasses of alkaline water or water with lemon juice.

A colonic has a profound cleansing effect on the body, and many people feel so good afterwards that they want to double their physical activity or work-out time (i.e. daily routine, jogging, etc.). **Caution is advised here,** for it can be overdone. Although light to moderate exercise is good if you are used to it, any strenuous activity should be avoided the day of your colonic session.

A light diet of fruits, vegetables, salads, soup, along with chicken or fish, should be followed for two days. Take care to avoid anything that causes gas (beans, cabbage, onions, etc.). Rich, heavy foods, flour products, spices and alcohol should also be avoided.

Although irrigation of the colon does not remove all of the intestinal bacteria, it is still often helpful to take some form of probiotics (beneficial bacteria) after-ward, such as acidophilus, to maintain a good bacterial balance. See Chapter 12, which covers supplements, for more on probiotics. There's information there on the Inner Body Bath Probiotic, which is available from my website, www. indiashealthyliving.com/.

FINDING A QUALIFIED COLON HYDROTHERAPIST

Before you get a colonic, take the time to do a little research, and don't let just anyone put their hands on you. A good resource for finding a reputable colon hydrotherapist is the website for the International Association of Colon Hydrotherapy (www.i-act.org). I-ACT establishes training standards and guide-lines. They are the certifying body for colon hydrotherapists around the world. They advise that you use an I-ACT board certified hydrotherapist who uses currently registered FDA equipment, disposable supplies, and filtered water. To find referred hydrotherapists in your area, go to the Referrals section of their website and search by zipcode, area code, city or state.

Chat on the phone with the colon hydrotherapist before you make an appointment. Ask about their education and level of certification. I-ACT has four levels. I am at the highest level, which is four. (There aren't very many people around who are at that level.) Also, how is their energy, their spirit? Will you want to develop a therapeutic relation-ship with this healer?

There are basically two types of colonics equipment: the closed tube or Closed System and the open basin or Open System. For photos of the different equipment, go to www.dotoloresearch. com/equipment.htm (for the closed system) and www.colonic.net (for the open system).

I use a *Closed System*. With this approach, the client is treated on a elevated platform that resembles a massage table. The client lies down, and we work with my colonics unit which has been plumbed into a wall cabinet to the right of the table. The unit has gauges and knobs that I control. With the patient on their side, I place the speculum, which is about the size of my thumb, by the place where it needs to be, and I have the client insert the lubricated speculum into their rectum. The patient becomes connected to the equipment once they have inserted the speculum. He or she often lies on their left side for the next 5 minutes, and the patient may then turn onto their back, right side or belly.

The speculum has two ports: one for inflow and the other for outflow. After the speculum is inserted, I direct the equipment to infuse fresh water through the correct hose into the client's colon. I also instruct the client to give me a signal when they feel that they've taken in as much water as they can handle. In addition, gauges on the device and my own observations of the body signals let me know when it's time to release the inserted water. For the client, this point feels similar to when you've really "got to go." When the time is right, I release the pressure and reverse the process, and the water and waste then travels back to the unit through the second hose. A viewing window in the unit allows the client and I to see the water and eliminated waste flowing through the equipment for disposal.

There is so much I can tell from what comes out. For instance, I can see if you are chewing your food well enough for the body to break it down. Sometimes food actually comes out the same way it went in, and that's not just corn but also slices of mushroom, chunks of potato with skin, pieces of pineapple, bits of nuts, and apple peel. I've even seen the labels that grocery stores put on fruits and vegetables (and that's not so unusual with my patients!). In addition to signs of a deficiency of chewing, I also look at the mucus that comes out, the consistency of the matter, the coloration of the stools.

Often I repeat the process of infusing and out-flowing water with a fresh batch of filtered water during the session. I also massage the client's abdomen during the colonic to help facilitate the loosening of the material on the walls of the colon. When we get waste out of your body, you can't help but feel better. *Life is good!*

With the *Open System* of Colon Hydrotherapy, the fiberglass table looks more like a recliner with a basin molded into it. A small tube for water inflow may be inserted by the therapist or the client into the rectum. There is then a flow of water into the colon. Once the colon is full, the rectal tube is removed and the client's own peristalsis moves the water and waste out. This outflow goes down through a drain in the bottom of the basin. The equipment is designed with an exhaust system so there is no odor involved.

As I mentioned, I prefer the closed system. And I always invite people to come over and see my facility before they lie down on the colonics table. If you live in our area or can travel to LA, give us a call at (323) 937-7300.

Understand that there is an art to colon hydrotherapy, so you want to select a therapist with experience. I have worked in this field for 17 years. An experienced hydrotherapist like myself will know how to administer a colonic in a way that will be most comfortable for you. I've had clients who became regulars with me after seeing another colon hydrotherapist they didn't want to see again, sometimes even after paying ahead for more sessions with the other practitioner. I specialize in making sure that my clients never walk away from my facility feeling like they've been violated, tortured or not educated. It is against my rules and ethics.

A BATH FOR YOUR COLON

During a colonic, your colon gets washed, and the colon hydrotherapist's job is to make sure it gets a good bath. However (this point bears repeating) only filtered water is used. Colonics expand and cleanse the colon pockets, tone and hydrate the colon, stimulate peristalsis, and help purify the blood and lymphatic system. A colonic is an energizing experience, and one's body is freed from the effects of its own toxicity following the procedure. I often marvel that someone thought to invent this process that is so supportive of optimal health.

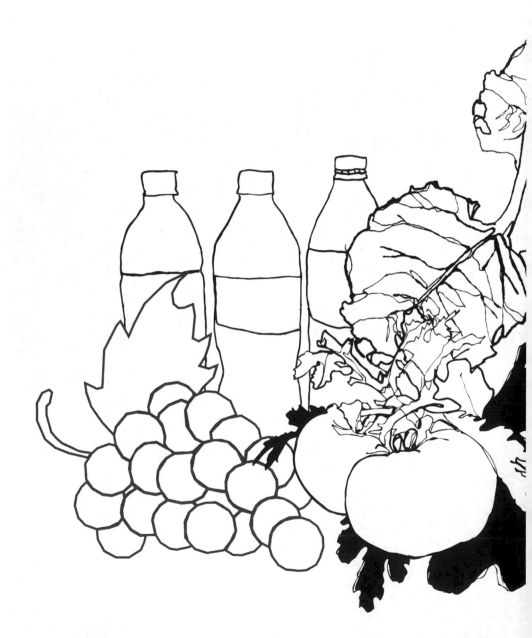

CHAPTER 4

Detox 101

YEARS AGO, THOMAS JEFFERSON predicted that the future physician would administer no medication but instead would interest his patients in healing naturally without surgery. This chapter will look at ways that you can support your body's natural healing capabilities through detoxification.

WE ARE A TOXIC SOCIETY

The World Health Organization reports that 90% of all chronic diseases are related to environmental factors, from pollution in the air, to toxins that come from what we eat, drink and wear. And let's not forget to mention toxins related to drugs – over-the-counter medications as well as doctors' prescriptions.

Junk food consumption has increased dramatically in the last few decades, bringing with it many chemicals. The average home today contains more chemicals than were found in a typical chemical lab at the turn of the century and more than 300 man-made chemicals have been found in human bodies. The full extent of the risk of these toxins to our bodies is unclear. What is clear, however, is that 50 years ago, through extensive processing, we began robbing nutrients from our foods. It's hard to determine what amounts of "diluted fortified nutrients" we are consuming.

OUR BODY'S ABILITY TO HEAL ITSELF

Toxic: Pertaining to, due to, or of the nature of a poison. (*Dorland's Illustrated Medical Dictionary*)

Toxicity: The quality of being poisonous, or the degree to which something is poisonous. (*Cambridge Dictionary of American English*)

Poison: A substance that causes illness or death if swallowed, absorbed or breathed into the body. (*Webster's Dictionary*)

Considering the level of toxicity today, it's fortunate that the human body is designed to detoxify on its own. At the same time, this magnificent Temple, the only one issued to us, requires internal harmony to work properly and to remain healthy. If you are an enemy of this body, the body will fight you. If you continue to take in more of the world's chemicals than the body is able to destroy and throw away, the body will perish. "Symptoms that last more than 120 days are a sign that the illness has passed from cell to cell and other body systems have become involved," notes author Brenda Watson, ND, in her book *Essential Cleansing for Perfect Health.*

The body detoxifies itself in various ways, including through the work of the lymphatic system, the skin, liver, lungs, kidneys, and the colon. The program in this book emphasizes working with the natural processes of detoxification, along with colonics and a lifestyle change. You'll find products that will support the body's detoxification processes in Chapter 12. At this point, let's look at some of the major detox systems in the human body.

THE LYMPHATIC SYSTEM

Your lymphatic system is your secondary circulatory system. Your primary circulatory system moves your blood, which is pumped by your heart to travel through the blood vessels. The lymphatic system doesn't have the luxury of a pump and requires your movement (exercise) to distribute your white blood cells. The white blood cells in the lymph are designed to nourish those parts of the body not fed by blood vessels, and they kill off harmful organisms and carry away the debris.

The key to keeping this important system running smoothly is *regular exercise.* Without regular exercise, your lymphatic fluid can become thick and toxic, and this system can develop blocks. "When the lymph slows down, the cells end up suspended in an acidic bath," says Dr. Robert Young in his book *The pH Miracle for Diabetes.* At that point, in no uncertain terms, a major cleanse is necessary.

The Skin

Your largest organ, the skin, can serve as an elimination channel for toxins when other systems fail, and you sometimes see the evidence in the form of rashes and other dermal eruptions. Certain toxins regularly pass out of the body through the skin when you sweat, and these can include heavy metals. Fat-soluble toxins, such as certain pesticides, can be purged by the body when

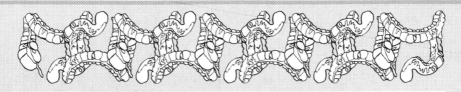

Diabetes & High Blood Pressure

Did you know that nearly 60% of people with high blood pressure have diabetes? Did you know that of those with diabetes, 80% are obese or overweight? Having diabetes doubles your chances of having a heart attack or heart-related problems including angina, stroke, triglycerides and high cholesterol. The body protects itself from excess acid (from excess sugars) – which can lead to holes in the blood vessels – by binding it with fats and minerals. Then the heart has to work harder to move blood to and from itself, pushing the same volume through narrowing blood vessels, which leads to elevated blood pressure. For more info on this, check out Dr. Robert Young's book, *The pH Miracle for Diabetes*.

sebaceous glands in the skin secrete sebum. Saunas and detox baths help us utilize the elimination pathways of the skin and the lymphatic system. Dry skin brushing also helps both systems process toxins.

The Liver
The second largest organ and a very active part of the body is the liver. It performs over 500 body functions. Toxins that enter the body from the intestinal tract are transported to the liver. The liver is constantly working to cleanse and filter 100 gallons of blood a day. The body cannot live without this organ.

The Lungs
The lungs filter every breath you take in. They are the breath of the body and require constant movement. When you exhale, the lungs release carbon dioxide as well as toxins in the form of gases. Mucus in the lungs captures other types of toxins, which are disposed of through coughing.

The Kidneys
There are a number of kidney concerns. Your kidneys come in a pair. Most people with mid-back pain on the right and left side of the spine never consider that these pains or discomforts may be related to their two kidneys. The kidneys, like the liver, filter blood and have the tricky task of differentiating between unwanted toxins and needed nutrients.

You may be 25 years old, eat correctly, exercise and perform all natural body care, essentially be a healthy person, yet the kidneys can build up thousands of stones and will eventually give you grief. The kidneys may be damaged by exposure to certain toxins, such as drugs. "It is so silly that kidney disease has become an epidemic in America, especially since it is so easy to prevent and so simple to heal," notes Dr. Richard Schulze. For information on Dr. Schulze's kidney formulas, go to the products section of my website http://indiashealthyliving.com/. and click on the link to his site.

Your Digestive System & Colon

Even with one bowel movement a day, there are still eight meals sitting in your digestive tract. If your digestive system is clean and healthy, it will produce good healthy bowel movements. A healthy digestive system and colon allows the important vitamins, minerals and nutrients to flow through and get absorbed by your entire body.

When foods are not chewed thoroughly and remain undigested in the colon, the colon then becomes crammed with hardened feces. Toxins from these feces get reabsorbed into the body. Yuck! Cleansing is essential.

Two of the most fundamental functions in life are to eat and to poop! It is a fact that too many people have been told and believe that it is OK to go for days without pooping. *Think again!* More importantly, if you have not pooped lately (in the last couple of days), you will may develop brain fog and have trouble thinking clearly! As far as I am concerned, there is nothing like a good bowel movement. In fact, pooping should be the highlight of your day … so relieving … so gratifying! Not pooping may make one irritable, angry, sluggish and mean, with a splash of evil. What's going on with you?

The entire alternative health community now agrees with Bernard Jensen's wisdom, that health begins in the colon. Keeping that colon healthy is the number one way to maintain health and prevent sickness.

COLON HYDROTHERAPY (CHT)

A colonic, also known as Colon Hydrotherapy (CHT), cleanses the colon as layers of buildup are removed. Then when one actually gets down to the mucous lining, real cleansing occurs.

While every person's diet, level of activity, and health differs, the average person would benefit from an initial series of three, five, and sometimes eight to ten colonics sessions before going on maintenance program (usually monthly, quarterly or bi-annually).

For more info on CHT, see Chapter 3: "Colon Hydrotherapy: What you'll want to know … How it works."

A DAILY DETOX ROUTINE

1. Drink water all day long.

Drink about 20 ounces of alkaline water or water with lemon upon rising in the morning. Those who can drink more: make that 30 ounces. (Avoid tap water; it contains heavy metals, chlorine, and is loaded with industrial waste.) Shake the water vigorously before drinking it. Get that water moving. The morning is one of the most vital times to be hydrating the body and the colon.

Throughout the day, drink plenty of water (half your body's weight in ounces). For example, if you weight 150 pounds, you should drink at least 75 ounces (150 divided by 2) of water. After the initial water upon awakening, drink two more 8-ounce glasses of water before noon. Drink your last 8-ounce glass of water just before going to bed at night. Drink your remaining ounces in the afternoon and evening. Without sufficient water, toxins are reabsorbed.

Acid is the breeding ground for disease. Consuming plenty of water is the best way to wash the acid out and then avoid putting more acid in.

The body is primarily made of water: 70% of the body's muscle is water, 25% of the body's fat is water, 75% of the body's brain is water, and 80% or more of the body's blood is water. Don't rely on soda or juice or alcohol to hydrate your body, and certainly not milk … rely on H_2O! Water regulates body temperature, cushions and protects the vital organs, aids in digestion in a big way, transports nutrients within cells, and DISPELS ACIDIC WASTES. Certainly, drinking plenty of water is critical to the health of your pancreas. You simply cannot ignore water.

Adults lose, on average, about 10 cups – roughly 2.4 liters – every day through sweating, exhaling (you can see your breath on a cool day or night), urinating, and bowel movements. Very active people lose even more, and most diabetics lose in excess of 4 liters a day through removing excess acids. At the very least, you need to replace what you're losing. *If you're only drinking enough to cover your losses, you won't provide enough water to flush out all those acids. And I repeat, acid is the breeding ground for all diseases.*

Alkaline is the opposite of acid; make sure your water is alkaline. Your meals should be at least 70% alkaline, with the remaining 30% acid. Disease cannot develop in an alkaline environment.

For a list of alkaline and acids foods, see Chapter 8, "It's Not a Diet, It's a Lifestyle."

2. Exercise regularly, including jumping on a rebounder or mini-trampoline.

Three to five minutes on a rebounder or mini-trampoline will stimulate the lymphatic system. A gentle motion is enough to stimulate lymph flow. When you move up and down on a rebounder, the force of gravity alternately pulls and then releases each cell, stimulating cellular fluid flow so that toxic material is flushed out. Nutrients are also absorbed. In addition, the valves in your lymphatic system open and shut when you rebound, pumping lymphatic fluid throughout your body. During this process, not only are toxins removed, but white blood cells (*killer cells that help fight infection*) are produced. You will also notice stimulation to the colon. Jumping on a rebounder, by far, is my favorite exercise.

Exercise benefits your heart, lungs and muscles. It also benefits the colon, and can make you more regular.

FROM ARTICLES.MERCOLA.COM

Other forms of exercise:

- Walking
- Jogging
- Swimming
- Jumping rope
- Bicycling
- Skiing
- Rowing
- Skating
- Cross-trainers
- Yoga
- Weight-training
- Aerobic exercise (high- and low-impact)
- Pilates
- Kettlebells

Passive stimulation of the lymph system:

- Saunas
- Lymphatic drainage (a type of massage that addresses the lymphatic system)
- Acupressure and acupuncture
- Dry skin brushing (self-massage)

3. Keep your stress at a minimum.

During acute stress, our body undergoes many physiological changes. For instance, the heart starts pounding to pump blood to our brain and is distributed from the brain to the body's many organs, the arms and legs. Of course, these days, stress often occurs not because something has come to eat us but because we've eaten some toxic foods. This causes the immune system to prepare to defend itself against the influx of toxins. Taking the immune system away from its normal routine is very unhealthy. It releases uric acid.

Unlike animals, humans react to stress in a chronic way. Stress stays with us longer than in animals and sometimes all our lives.

When we experience stress of any kind – including but not limited to mental stress, emotional stress, and physical stress – energy (along with blood, enzymes and oxygen) is diverted away from the digestive tract: results, constipation.

4. Brushing one's teeth (and flossing) is an essential part of the cleansing routine.

There is a lot of evidence that whenever there is a serious disease, there may be a problem in the mouth. For instance, Dr. William Nordquist, BS DMD MS discusses the possibility that heart disease could be connected to gum disease in his book, *The Stealth Killers: Is Oral Spirochetosis the Missing Link in the Dental and Heart Disease Labyrinth?* Spirochetes are a potent bacteria involved in gingivitis (gum disease).

Brush with a *natural* toothpaste after meals, and remember to floss on a regular basis.

5. Aim for six small meals a day.

Eating small meals more often helps to raise your metabolism. It also keeps your blood levels more even, which keeps your energy up. In addition, you won't feel as starved when you do eat.

Here are some nutritious foods to include: nuts, raisins, fruit, salads, soups and herbal teas.

Tips:

a. Eat five almonds, *not* the whole can or bag.

b. Buy the small snack-size boxes of raisins.

c. Squeeze natural lemon over sliced fruit and eat sl-o-o-o-o-o-w.

d. Try soy yogurt with granola if lactose intolerant.

6. Stay away from fast food!

(Discussed in greater detail in Chapter 8, "It's Not a Diet, It's a Lifestyle.")

Junk foods have little or no nutritional value. Fast food is dead food. If you're interested in dying sooner or causing sickness, then, by all means, help yourself. But fast food and this program cancel one another out!

Through the process of detoxification and eating more nutritiously, you can access the keys to healing and regeneration.

Other tips:

• Take time out of the day to clear your mind for 10 minutes (to de-stress).

• Exercise daily for no less than 45 minutes.

• Brush your teeth twice daily with natural toothgel (see the "Walking My Talk" chapter [Chapter 6] for my dental health regimen).

• Keep peppermint and or ginger tea handy in case of queasiness or nausea. (See the next chapter, "The Healing Crisis vs. The Disease Crisis.")

• Manage your health; take your blood pressure and monitor your sugar levels daily. (Once again, I remind you to *Manage your health, not a disease!*)

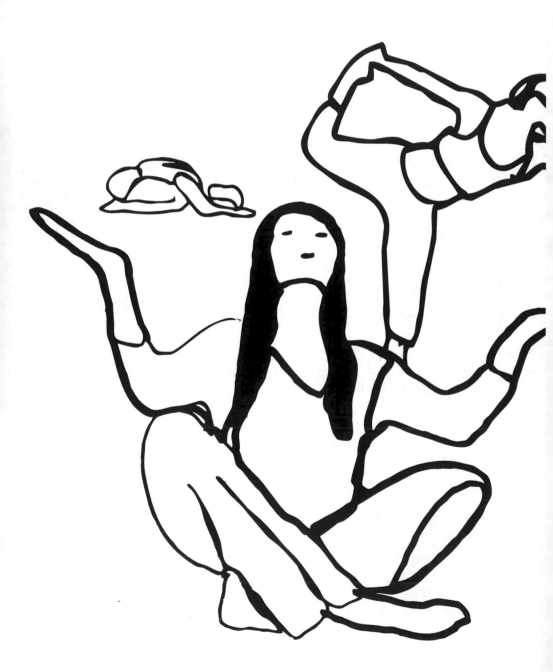

CHAPTER 5

The Healing Crisis Versus the Disease Crisis

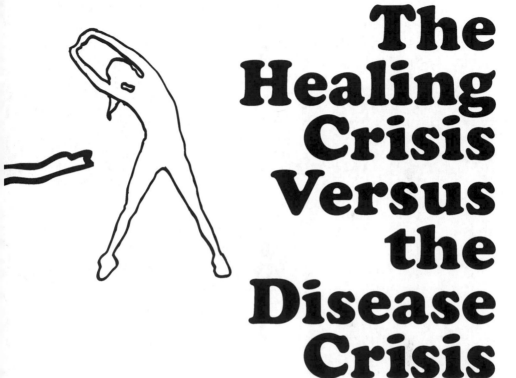

WHEN YOU BEGIN YOUR DETOXIFICATION program, you must clean the colon thoroughly. Eat the right combination of foods and, just as important, health-supporting and healing foods. Exercise and maintain a good spiritual attitude. Keep stress at a minimum in your life (stress alone can kill you!) and get sufficient rest. As I have been emphasizing, it is essential to drink sufficient amounts of water. When you make these changes, you will begin to produce positive effects in your body and build a strong immune system.

A brisk walk at least 45 minutes a day can reduce the risk of cancer by 40%. Eating less red meat and processed/fast foods (for instance, bologna, hot dogs and sausage [pork, beef, chicken, turkey sausage, whatever!] will reduce the risk of cancer by 35%. Cut the bacon and quesadillas, **please.** There is no question that men must cut down or eliminate altogether their intake of burgers and particularly males in the African-American community. It's a killer the amount of burgers you guys gulp down. Aim for no processed foods at all.

THE CIRCULATORY SYSTEM

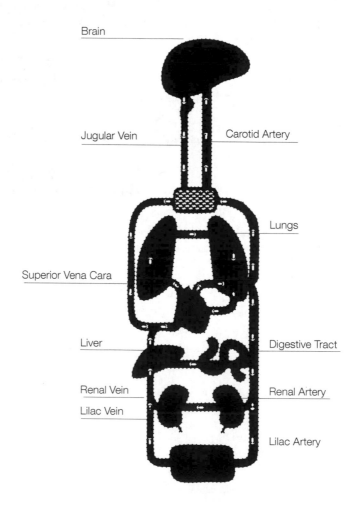

Brain

Jugular Vein

Carotid Artery

Lungs

Superior Vena Cara

Liver

Digestive Tract

Renal Vein

Renal Artery

Lilac Vein

Lilac Artery

THE BIG FLUSH

As you read in the last chapter, the function and efficiency of some of our organs, the lymphatic system, and other channels of elimination are designed to move and push out toxic waste:

The Skin from Perspiration

The Lungs from Respiration

The Kidneys through Urination

The Colon though Elimination …

The heart circulates blood, which carries nutrients (food) and oxygen to all the cells of the body. And the blood carries away waste products so that they can be removed from the body (after being filtered by the kidneys). Without access to the blood, cells and body tissues die.

These organs and systems will function far more proficiently once cleansed.

As you go through the process of removal and cleansing of excess waste, some discomforts may take place. Consider the dormant waste in the colon from a lifestyle of consuming non-nutritious foods. Years of waste that's been tucked away for a long time, minding its own business. And along comes "the flush," a daily poop, eating right, supporting supplements that are health-building and body-healing. Indeed, instead of packing, accumulating and building a swamp of waste (as most bodies are doing), your body is letting go, eliminating, and ultimately healing and rejuvenating.

As it should.

The body is designed to ingest, digest, assimilate and eliminate, not hurry up, gobble up, bloat up and back up. Your body was not designed to capture waste and store it like a cesspool. Instead, it's made to use foods for fuel and dump what it does not use, need or want in the form of waste on *a daily basis.*

As you are going through a detoxification program, toxins will exit the body any way they can. Accumulated toxins have lain submerged for years, and the minute you begin to shake them up, these toxins will try to leave – *all at once.* As efficient as the body is, it's not easy for it to adjust within 24 hours to handle this bombardment of poisons that are now ripping and roaring out. In most cases, these toxins have accumulated, and they've been packed in over a period of *many* years. Are you getting the picture? They cannot all come out at one time but they will try, and you will feel it. What you're feeling is the HEALING CRISIS, also known as BURN-OFF!

SYMPTOMS OF THE HEALING CRISIS

As waste leaves the body, there may be some minor discomforts – such as headaches, unpleasant sensations in the stomach (queasiness), and gas. Your body is readjusting to proper balancing and a new chemistry. Your appetite may alter; additionally, you may get nauseous and/or vomit. There may be feelings of faintness and weakness. There will be some weight loss at first and, indeed, men will respond more noticeably than the women in that department. As you begin to eliminate waste through detoxification, it may seem as

the b
desig
to ing

ody is

med

est...

though a cold is coming on. In fact, a common cold is simply an expression of the body's attempt to clean house (get rid of toxins or germs). If at that point of your detox, you try to suppress the cold with drugs or medication of any kind, the toxins will indeed go back into the bloodstream only to be hoarded and accumulate somewhere else. *NO FUN!* You could even have symptoms of influenza that may turn flu-like for several days to a week, depending on the level of toxins in the system.

You may notice a scratchy throat, mucus and other signs of waste (from accumulated rancid fats, devitalized [processed] and denatured foods [fast foods]) starting to move out; cleansing and purifying is happening! *This is the burn-off.* You will realize the lasting benefits of your change in eating habits as soon as your body readjusts to its proper balance.

For those of you who have been food junkies for YEARS and/or are chock-full of waste (you know who you are), it may take a little longer to realize the trade-up. Remember the healing crisis is temporary … However, if progressive body condition(s) have always entered the picture (for instance, maybe if you were a sickly child or developed pathological conditions as you aged), achievement of balance will be harder and take longer. The key is not to wait until it's too late. You are probably well aware that as you get older, the body is always in ever-changing stages … For instance, your metabolism slows. As a matter of fact, the production of certain nutrients (that the body produced naturally when you were younger) slows down or ceases altogether.

HOW LONG WILL THE HEALING CRISIS LAST?

The longer the deficiencies, poisons and need for purifications have existed, the more prevalent the healing crisis response is likely to be. Not in all cases but in many, you may feel worse before you feel better. However, again, it's only temporary and very short-term. The gauge for complete healing reads like this: **for every year you've caused your body distress and disease, it will take a month to repair …** *You do the math.*

This repair requires *consistency.* Your body doesn't understand iffy. It doesn't understand that this day you're on, and this day you're off … **consistency is the key.**

All your body needs from you, to heal, is balance. It cannot achieve balance if you are the enemy! When there is imbalance, the body must work harder to keep you alive, healthy, whole, sane and happy. **The healing crisis is a hard-working effort of every organ in the body to eliminate waste products and establish the balance point for rejuvenation and to stop degeneration.** Every organ in the body works in harmony with one another to establish and maintain this balance. Take the enemy out of the picture (YOU, MY FRIEND) and the body will heal itself – with your help, of course.

By constantly eating the foods the body does not want, need or can handle, you are continuously causing a slow and

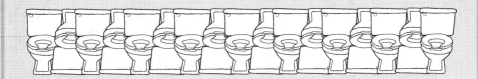

HOW TO RIDE OUT THE HEALING CRISIS

1. **SLEEP.** At this time, the body needs rest. When you sleep, the body rejuvenates.

2. **BREATHE.** Breathing is one of the least appreciated human functions, according to the Somax Sports Performance Institute (www.somaxsports.com). They say that "constriction in breathing can cause poor skin tone, fatigue, pain, premature senility, poor athletic performance, osteoporosis and heart attacks." **SCARY!** Pay attention to your breathing, and see if you breathe fully down into your abdomen. Many people are shallow-breathers. If you are one of these folks, then consciously practice breathing more deeply until it becomes a habit.

3. **REMEMBER TO BREATHE DEEPLY DURING EXERCISE.** One of the most important benefits of exercise is blowing off carbon dioxide. As carbon dioxide accumulates in our lungs, less oxygen gets to the brain. Deep breathing sends fresh oxygen to the brain. Since our brain runs on oxygen and sugar, not having enough can lead to fatigue and fuzzy thinking. We blow off the carbon dioxide when we get moving, and this is why we feel less fatigued after exercising.

4. **POOP REGULARLY.** I personally believe that pooping is the most unappreciated human function, even more than breathing. But I digress ...

5. **KEEP DRINKING YOUR WATER.** And plenty of it with lemon (lemon helps quicken the removal of waste or unwanted toxins from the body).

continuous buildup of wastes and breakdown of tissue.

WHO ARE YOU FOOLING?

Don't think that you can maintain a healthy existence by doing all the right things, but you're continuing to drink three cups of coffee daily ... the Kidneys are pissed off! Although you may not see it immediately, this behavior will eventually take its toil.

If you work out five days a week but are over-weight because you eat like a farm animal, the heart can only take so much of that stress. Or you maintain good habits but cannot kick sucking poisons into your lungs (smoking) ...

diges
accu
late
elim

st,

mu-

nd

nate

the Lungs are exhausted, not to mention full of exhaust. And how about when you eat two times a day but only poop once every other day. Guess what? Through the colon all things must pass ... and when you clog up that bad boy (the colon), you can't even think straight (the brain is doing the moon walk and you don't know if you're coming or going). The body knows you're trying to poison it, and it's sending out all the signals for you to get yourself under control. Listen to the body's language, its symptoms. What are some of those symptoms? Try anything from foul breath to major headaches. It's time to listen. Indeed, you are slowly moving towards a **degeneration crisis.**

DEGENERATION CRISIS

You have five eliminatory organs: the colon, skin, lungs, liver and kidneys. All your organs begin excess dumping of waste during a **healing crisis,** not during a degeneration or *disease crisis.*

During a **disease crisis** or degeneration of the body, the organs of elimination will **accumulate** waste. It holds on and builds up waste. Any buildup in the body is a disease, from a boil under the arm to fluid on the lungs. It's because you've accumulated and retained waste buildup in that area or path of elimination.

You know a disease crisis as your body communicates with you. During this crisis, you may witness constipation, glandular enlargement, joint pains, and mucous buildup and so on; any

accumulation in the body is a sign of disease. Your body is saying or screaming:

"EXCUSE ME! FIX IT! STOP DOING IT! OR GIVE ME WHAT I NEED!"

In order for the cells to renew health to the body, all excess waste *must go.* When witnessing a fever and/or a sore throat, it *appears* to be a disease crisis. Actually your body is trying to rid itself of waste and foreign matter, or kill germs and unfriendly bacteria. At this point, it is a healing crisis!

WHAT HAPPENS WITH A CONSCIOUS DETOX PROGRAM

For some, usually you major red-meat eaters, the experience of going through a healing crisis will seem a lot like having the disease or illness itself. I've had clients actually go to the Emergency Room during a healing crisis. This is rare but that's how bad you may feel. The ER doctor takes blood and determines there are toxins in the blood. *Hello!*

Do Not! ... I repeat, Do Not think that your butt is on fire when you're doing a conscious detox program and your body is trying to clean itself. The Old Doc at the ER is just standing by waiting to issue the proverbial pill.

There is a distinct difference between the healing crisis and a disease or degeneration crisis. Those differences are elimination with healing as opposed to accumulation or buildup of waste with

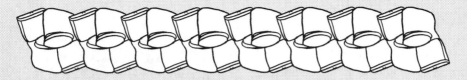

ALLERGIC REACTIONS

If any allergic-type of reaction occurs, chances are that it was caused by the hydrochloric acid in the stomach (which may be deficient) and/or the adrenal glands and liver could be in a state of dysfunction (not working properly).

AN ALLERGIC-TYPE REACTION MAY SHOW IN THE FORM OF

1. Extreme gas

2. You may break out in a rash if you have weak or sensitive skin.

3. There may be a metallic taste in your mouth, causing funky breath.

4. There may be symptoms of a cold or the flu, such as excess mucus.

5. You may feel sluggish or tired.

6. Headaches

7. Joint pains

8. Nausea or vomiting

Your body has but one innate memory and that is **the will to heal**. It is the will of every cell, every tissue in your body, to cleanse and purify or throw off toxic material.

REVIEW
WHEN YOU BEGIN YOUR DETOX PROGRAM YOU MUST

1. Clean the colon thoroughly and all your other organs of elimination.

2. Eat the health-supportive/body-healing foods.

3. Eat the right combination of foods.

4. Exercise.

5. Maintain a good TRUE spiritual attitude ... To begin to produce positive changes in your body, you must act on your faith – not just speak of it.

6. Walk at least 45 minutes a day. Or do other exercises for that period of time.

7 Eat less red meat and processed/fast foods. Try cutting them out altogether for one month while detoxing. You may never return to them!

8. Drink one-half your body weight in ounces of water daily, the first 20 to 30 ounces upon rising in the morning, two more before noon, and the last bottle or glass just before bed. Drink more in the afternoon and evening.

9. Take a good detox colon cleanser along with a good probiotic (see Chapter 12 for my suggestions).

10. Get regular colonics or take daily enemas, if fasting.

degeneration. The price you will have to pay for this short time (one to five days) of healing crisis far outweighs the misery and agony of a disease when the body begins to break down faster than it can heal itself. NOW, YOU ARE IN A DISEASE CRISIS!

Let's just give it a name ... or a diagnosis. With the healing crisis, the body is consistently throwing out waste. With the disease crisis, the body holds on to waste, and damages tissue and cells, as things continue to degenerate. One thing for sure is evident: you are not as efficient in the poop department during a disease crisis. That's right ... This is the time when a condition known as Constipation will occur!

The healing crisis ordinarily lasts for a short period of time, about one to five days, starting with slight pain and discomfort that may become more severe until the point of complete expulsion has been reached. During this time, there is an absence of appetite. One should follow the body's natural cravings or follow the simple rule of eating live foods: "If it **rots or spoils, eat it (but eat it before it does)."**

Your body has but one innate memory and that is the will to heal.

THE BODY DOESN'T KNOW HOW TO DIE.

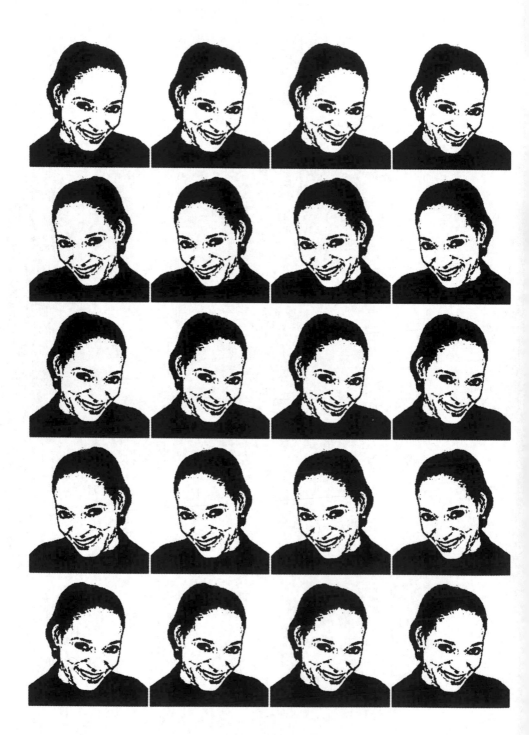

CHAPTER 6

A Typical Day of Walking My Talk

WHEN I DO RADIO INTERVIEWS, there's one thing people always want to know more about – **my daily routine.** My editor Robin and I decided to cover this routine in an interview for this sixth chapter. I don't expect you to follow everything that I do each day, but look for some habits that you could start to incorporate into your own life. Other chapters offer additional ideas for positive lifestyle changes.

RQ: Tell me about your typical day. How does it start?

IH: For the most part, I get a great night's sleep. I sleep so good, it's scary. So I wake up feeling really refreshed. I typically get 7 to 8 hours of sleep.

The first thing I do is drink my water. I get up about 5 o'clock and I drink about 20 ounces, straight down, of the alkaline water. And then I go back to bed for half an hour.

At that time in the morning, your body has been fasting for 8 hours. So it's ready for anything that comes in. The first thing I put in there is the alkaline water. It goes straight to the colon. As the water is percolating in my body, I begin to hear growling … the bowel sounds.

RQ: How long does it take you to drink that amount of water?

IH: Just 30 seconds. I drink it straight down.

I recommend people to drink 20 to 30 ounces. Sometimes I do more. But for sure, drink 20 ounces. Because I am drinking alkaline water, it hydrates the body and the bowel faster than clean regular water.

I have the alkaline water ready in a bottle on my bedstand, and it has already been measured out the night before. And it's room temperature. You don't want anything cold going in your body, especially first thing in the morning … it just constricts things.

Also, before I even get out of bed for the day, I take my blood pressure. I have my blood pressure cup at the edge of the bed, and I pull it out and I stick it on my arm and press the button. Then I lie there for the few minutes that it takes for the blood pressure cup to generate the reading. And then, *voilà* – 116 over 69. It was beautiful again this morning. I love seeing that every day.

I take my blood pressure before going to bed at night as well. Readings of under 120 for the top number and below 80 for the bottom number are considered healthy or normal readings. I consistently get those good numbers.

RQ: What comes next?

IH: After that, I get up and right away I run the bath water.

As the bath water is running, I put my ingredients in there – I get my slush going. I add hydrogen peroxide, Epsom salt, and some alkaline water to the bath water.

The hydrogen peroxide actually pulls waste to the surface of the skin when I soak in the tub. And it helps push the waste out. That's why my skin stays so smooth and clear without having to use much soap or any lotions.

Also, I prepare my mouthwash and get everything ready to brush my teeth after I have my breakfast.

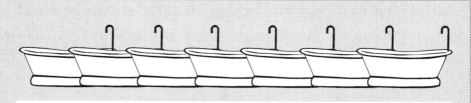

Formula for India's Detox Bath Slush

1 gallon of the Kangen water™ (Helps alkalinize all the water.)
1 cup Hydrogen Peroxide
1 cup of Epsom Salt
1 cup of Baking Soda
India also runs her Water Ozonator for about 15-20 minutes.
(The Ozonator can be purchased at www.superiorhealthproducts.com.)

In addition to mixing the mouthwash, I also put bentonite clay, activated charcoal and peppermint oil in a small cup to dip my toothbrush and toothpaste in after breakfast. The clay/charcoal combination helps to pull out the unwanted bacteria from the mouth, and the peppermint oil is for the taste as well as it being an anti-viral and an anti-bacterial.

Then I roll on the floor with my dog for a minute because she needs her special attention.

RQ: Of course she does.
IH: And she insists.

RQ: What's your dog's name.
IH: Her name is Mica. She's a standard German Schnauzer. Grey/black in color.

When the tub is full, I turn off the water. And I attach the Ozonator to the water. I bubble up the water with the Ozonator to zap the water..

RQ: Why do you use the Ozonator?
IH: It zaps all of the impurities in the water and pulls them out.

RQ: How did you discover this?
IH: First of all, I refuse to take a shower because when you do, you're breathing that chlorine into your lungs. And that's dangerous.

Unless you have a filter on your shower head.

I've done so much research and investigation to figure out all the natural things that people can do to keep the body healthy ... taking care of one's self without having to spend a lot of unnecessary money. I'm my own guinea pig for the most part. My philosophy is: "There is no better physician on this earth for your body than you!"

RQ: Do you bathe before breakfast?
IH: No I let the Ozonator run, and Mica and I both go downstairs, and I cook the oatmeal.

As the oatmeal is cooking, I'm doing my stretching. I might hop on the rebounder for a while and work my arms with Kettlebells. Or do a little Pilates as Mica steps outside to do her business.

RQ: Sounds like you're not using instant oatmeal ...
IH: No, nothing precooked from a box, can or bag if I can help it.

RQ: What kind of oatmeal do you eat?
IH: It's the 5-minute Quaker Oatmeal.

RQ: Why oatmeal?
IH: It's soluble fiber. Soluble fiber tends to absorb the toxins in so they can be moved out of the body.

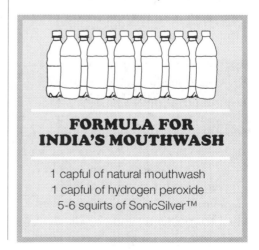

FORMULA FOR INDIA'S MOUTHWASH

1 capful of natural mouthwash
1 capful of hydrogen peroxide
5-6 squirts of SonicSilver™

And it's great with cholesterol. My cholesterol is beautiful.

I make enough oatmeal for my husband and myself. And I add raisins, agave nectar and sea salt.

RQ: How much of each?
IH: Half a teaspoon of sea salt, 2 tablespoons of agave, and about ¼ cup of raisins.

Boy, is that good.

RQ: Is there any coffee in this breakfast routine?
IH: Heck, no. Just water in the morning. Later, I have the Rooibos Red African Tea when I get to work.

When the oatmeal is cooked, I traipse back upstairs and sit in the bathwater. And I eat my oatmeal in the bath and catch up on some of my reading.

I never rush in the morning. *Never.* It's too much stress. I think: *If I have to go anywhere, like work, I give myself plenty time.*

I sit in the tub, and I wash with Dr. Bronner's natural bar soap. I like the peppermint Bronner's, because it's tingly.

RQ: Sounds like a great bath.
IH: Yes. And after that great bath, I take out my supplements. I have a whole drawer just for supplements. When my husband built the room, he made it so that I'd have a vanity drawer for all my makeup. But I use it for my supplements. I'm up to 18 different supplements a day that I take. For instance, I had arthritis in my thumb. The thumb was inflamed to the point that anything

that touched it made me want to slap it. And I have real serious cases of arthritis in my family to the point where some of them are in wheelchairs. Taking glucosamine made a big difference for me. So little by little, I started adding more things. (See Chapter 12 for more info on supplements.)

I take the supplements as I'm putting on my face, so to speak. For my makeup, I use all natural stuff. More and more, I use Jason beauty products, including their natural cosmetics. I love their products to the point where slowly but surely it looks like everything is becoming Jason. And I refer other people to Jenson's as well. You can find the Jason Natural Cosmetics online and they carry it at many health foods stores as well.

So there is hair gel, toothpaste, lip balm … just about everything that I do is from Jason, except the mascara which I purchase at Whole Foods. It's also natural.

And then I use a natural press powder from Sally Hansen. The Cornsilk natural powder comes in a little compact with a mirror. It's transparent, and you put it on, and it absorbs the oil.

Shall I talk about my elimination? I haven't talked about that yet, have I?

RQ: Sure. You are the Poop Police, after all.
(We both laugh.)
IH: Usually after I've had my oatmeal, I am ready for a bowel movement.

I make a bowel movement that is so phenomenal … I'm so proud of my bowel movements in the morning. I must stand and salute it.

I wonder at times, where did that come from? Certainly not me. It looks like a Great Dane just left something behind.

I don't eat as much as it appears when that comes out. But one thing a lot of people are not aware of is that 70-80% of your poop is water! So if you're not drinking your water, you're going to have dry constipated turds!

That is what's causing a lot of diseases. Like Diverticulosis, which is inflamed pockets along the intestines, a condition that can lead to all kinds of other problems ... I could go on and on and on. There's also the straining, and the hemorrhoids, and a host of other things that will crop up. People are not drinking enough water! And we're talking about water, not tea or coffee. The body needs water.

It only takes me a few seconds to make that much massive poop. Sometimes I like to sit there a while longer just to read.

RQ: Tell me about the food you take to work.
IH: When I'm dressed, I go downstairs, and snatch food from the refrigerator that I'm going to eat throughout the day. It's mostly fruit, and I'll usually have a bag of salad.

RQ: What kind of fruit?
IH: Today, for instance, I have watermelon, a white peach, an apple, an orange and sliced pineapple. And I eat that all day. At some point, I'll put a salad in between the fruit ... it depends on how I feel. That serving of oatmeal keeps me going. But it wouldn't for most people.

RQ: Do you have one serving of oatmeal in the morning?
IH: Yes.

RQ: And you just have the fruit and salad off and on throughout the day?
IH: Because I'm usually very busy. In between my clients, I maybe have a 15 minute window. So I'll eat something ... if I'm not on the phone returning a phone call.

RQ: Do you take a lunch break?
IH: I go straight through. People always wonder how I'm able to get through a day like this. And I think it's a combination of mental stability, good physical structure ... and getting regular exercise.

RQ: So is there anything else that you do at work that's different besides your diet?
IH: Well, we have a small gym here at the clinic, so occasionally I'll go in there.

If I'm working on really large people, I'll go into the gym between each one. Sometimes I'll have three large male clients in a row with appointments for colon hydrotherapy. So at the gym, I'll do strength-training with weights, some Pilates, and jump on the rebounder. I'll pump up my muscles.

In between clients, I also refresh myself and the room with essential oils. I make up my own mix ... in a spray bottle. I use alkaline water and oils such as sage, lavender, and a combination of peppermint and valor. Valor is a mix by Young Living Essential Oils. It contains coconut oil, spruce, rosewood and frankincense.

RQ: How long are your sessions with your clients?
IH: No more than 45 minutes.

RQ: How many clients do you usually see in a day?
IH: I average six clients a day during the week. Sometimes it's more.

RQ: You don't work at night ... you usually finish by 5 pm?
IH: I'm usually finished by 5 and I am out by 6. Before I leave, I set up for the next day. And return the phone calls that I get.

Then, at the end of the day, I gather up all my stuff and carry it all home. I'm in between at least four books at a time. Most of them are reference guides for the things that I wish to research..

And then there's my laptop computer, and sometimes I am dragging two laptops. One I don't hook up to the Internet. I just write with it. I drive 33 miles home, in the traffic, I am eating nuts ... almonds, raw. I may have one of my pieces of fruit that I have left over. And I have my alkaline water. And that is my snack activity to take me home. Sometimes it fills me up so that I don't have to eat dinner. In that case, I'm done for the day with food.

RQ: What do you do when you get home?
IH: First, I walk the dog, and I give her dinner. The walk is maybe 25 minutes.

And I always try to get the walk in as soon as I get home. So after I'm finished with the dog, and I get her all squared away, I fix dinner for my husband. He calls himself "the Big Dog."

A typical meal would be like last night ... an ear of corn, some broccoli, cauliflower, lightly steamed, and shrimp. Steamed shrimp.

RQ: Does your husband have any kind of a carb, like rice?
IH: Sometimes because he just loves the rice. But only if he prepares it. I'm not cooking it. So he'll prepare it, and he'll have rice with his meal.

He'll have a soda, or water, or juice. He loves juice.

RQ: Do you exercise before or after this meal?
IH: Sometimes I'm doing it in-between cooking. If I put something on that requires a little time on the stove or in the oven, I go upstairs and do my exercises.

There is more of the rebounder. More of the Pilates. And more of the Kettlebell weights.

Sometimes I'm listening to the news or the radio while I'm exercising. Catching up with the current affairs.

RQ: How do you spend the time after dinner?
IH: I take my laptops and I set up my second office in the family room. On the table, I have all my books and other things. I unload the carrier that I dragged in, and I hook up the

computers, and I have at it for another couple hours. And I try to avoid all other communication. I usually leave my cell phone in the car unless I'm expecting an important phone call.

I look at my schedule for the radio broadcast. See who is going to be on. Make sure that I have someone lined up for the next visit.

I read my emails. If I'm going to do a lecture, sometimes I am coordinating it with whoever is going to be doing it with me. The co-lecturer, or whatever.

Sometimes I'm preparing to give a lecture, like the one I gave recently to the National Youth Leadership Forum at UCLA.

RQ: What time do you go to sleep?
IH: I'm in bed by 9:45. Before that, I may sit by the window with the dog for 5 minutes before I go to bed.

Then, in bed, I watch *Seinfeld* as I get ready to sleep and very often I laugh out loud.

RQ: What are your weekends like?
IH: My Saturdays are usually a little slower than my other workdays. I'll start at 9 and I'll end at 1 or at my office.

I spend 3 to 5 hours at the Cerritos for the Performing Arts (my fun job) where I work as a Facility Assistant. And Sunday is a girl's day out.

First I walk the dog.

Then Mica and I make the rounds. We go to the car wash, the bank, the store.

My favorite stop on Sunday is to the Long Beach Farmer's Market, which is open from 9 am to 2 pm. It's held in the parking lot of the Long Beach Marina. I try to just buy produce in season. One of the nice things about this market is that it's within a half mile of Whole Foods and Trader Joe's. So I can just go from one to the other.

Sunday afternoon I sit at the computer, and catch up on things or church or the Cerritos Center for The Performing Arts.

RQ: What kinds of social events do you and your husband enjoy together?
IH: My husband is a big jazz buff. He knows all the bands and has a big music collection. He also likes to play the piano. A couple Sundays back, we went to a jazz brunch together.

We also will get tickets to the Cerritos Center for an evening out with friends. Other times, we just go out for dinner.

RQ: Anything else that you'd like to add?
IH: The amazing thing about all these habits is that I now look younger than I did years earlier. In fact, the other day family came by to visit, and I was looking at myself in an old video. My grandson is 14 years old now and he was only one at the time the video was shot. I look younger today than I did back in 1997! I feel better, too. Better choices make such a difference!

CHAPTER 7

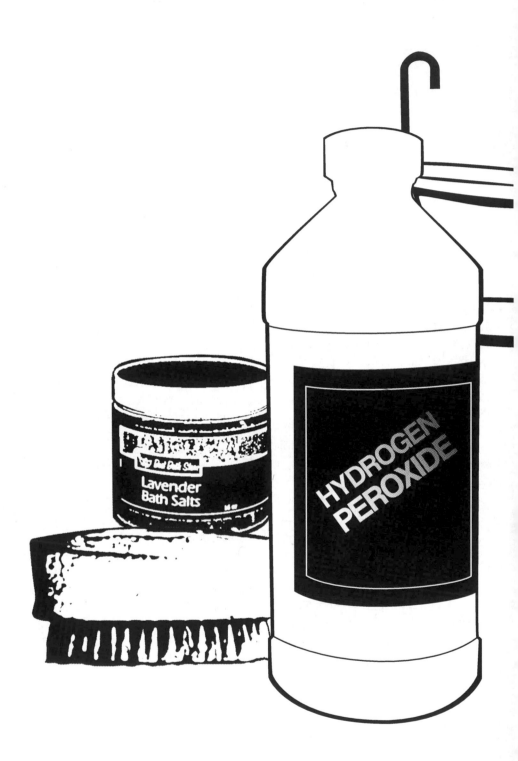

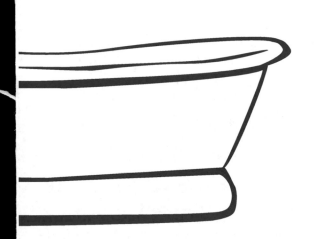

Detox Bath Time

Part of detoxing is bathing the body. Remember, your skin is your largest organ. Like other major organs (the liver, lungs, kidney and colon), the skin also eliminates.

So when going through a detox of any kind, you must also detox the skin and each of its layers.

Begin with Dry Skin Brushing

Dry brush the skin with a natural bristle brush to remove particles and debris from the pores (i.e. lotions, body oils, dead skin and whatever has landed on you from the air). **Yuk.** Look for a natural bristle brush with a long handle so you can reach your back.

Brush in circular motions, up from the feet over the legs toward the heart. From out-stretched arms, continue over the fingers and up the arms toward the heart. Brush the torso and the back as well, again toward the heart. Don't scratch yourself to death – just brush enough to stimulate the lymphatic system and remove the dead free-loaders.

Background on Epsom Salt

Epsom salt is a pure chemical compound (magnesium sulfate) in crystal form that gently exfoliates the skin and smoothes rough patches. Dissolved in a bath, Epsom salt is absorbed through the skin to replenish the body's level of magnesium. Studies indicate that this may help to relieve stress in a number of ways, including:

- Raising the body's level of serotonin, a mood-elevating chemical within the brain that creates feelings of well-being and relaxation.
- Offsetting excess levels of adrenaline generated by pressure and stress. Magnesium ions relax the body and reduce irritability by lowering the effects of adrenaline.
- Helping to regulate the electrical functions that spark through miles of nerves.
- Lowering blood pressure.

Researchers have found that magnesium also increases energy and stamina by encouraging the production of ATP (adenosine triphosphate), the energy packets made in the cells.

Studies have shown other possible benefits from the *magnesium* in Epsom salt:

- Improving sleep and concentration by reducing stress.
- Helping the muscles and nerves to function properly.
- Regulating the activity of 325+ enzymes.
- Helping to prevent hardening of the arteries and blood clots.

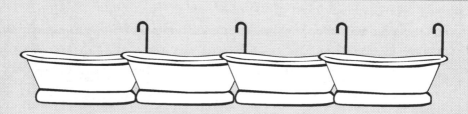

The Basic Formula

As I mentioned in the "Walking My Talk" chapter, I begin every day with a detox bath. Here's an easy formula that you can use for your own detox bath:

- 1 cup Epsom Salt
- 1 cup Baking Soda
- 1 cup Hydrogen Peroxide

If you have access to alkaline water, add a gallon of it to your bathwater. This will help to make all the water more alkaline.

The bath water should be hot, but not so hot that it would be unsafe for your body. Bathe for approximately 30 minutes, and then shower.

This bath acts as a magnet. It pulls toxins out of your body and into the bath water.

Aim for taking this detox bath twice a week, if you are unable to do it daily. Soon you will start to look better, feel better, and have more energy.

- Making insulin more effective.
- Reducing inflammation to relieve pain and muscle cramps.
- Improving oxygen use.

Below are some of the benefits from the *sulfates* in Epsom salt. (Note: You may have heard some negative things about sulfates, which are actually mineral salts containing sulfur. Sulfates have a different affect on the body when they are ingested in food, than when they are absorbed into the skin during a bath.)

- Flushing toxins.
- Improving the absorption of nutrients.
- Helping form joint proteins, brain tissue, and mucin proteins (used for lubrication and mineralization).

Joe Matusic, a pediatrician in Charleston, West Virginia, notes that Epsom salts can soothe just about anything that itches or burns the skin. "It's inexpensive, readily available, and an old-time remedy that works," he remarks.

An Alternative Detox Bath

Here is another formula that can be used when the small follicles of the skin are clogged up with grime and/or chemicals. For instance, this would be a good detox bath for a man who works with oil.

This detox bath also helps to destroy parasites and fungus, in addition to detoxifying the body.

The formula:

- 2 boxes baking soda
- 2 cups lemon-scented chlorine bleach

Again, use hot water that is at a safe temperature. Bathe for approximately 30 minutes, then shower.

Note: **Children with eczema**, ages 6 months to 17 years, should bathe for 20 minutes only – also in hot water – followed by a shower.

Splashingly Good

Why not find some time to soak in a detox bath? Besides the health benefits, a little pampering of yourself can't hurt. It will also be an opportunity to *slow down*.

"Detox baths are wonderfully healing."
~ Annie B. Bond

"I think a lot of contemplation happens in bathtubs. It does for me. Nothing like a hot bath to ease the tension and think about what's going to happen next."
~ Sarah McLachlan

"Taking a bath is just another way to play."
~ Adine Cathey

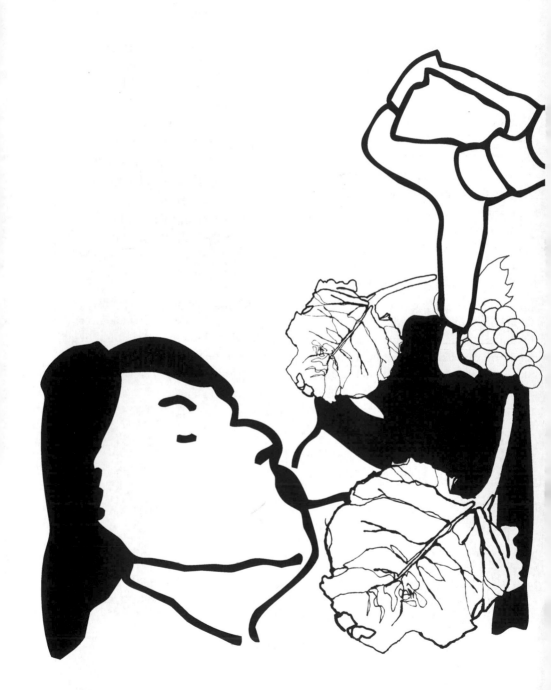

CHAPTER 8

It's Not Just a Diet, It's a Lifestyle Change

WHEN IT COMES to balancing out the body with food, I like to emphasize this theme: **too much is unnecessary, and too little is inefficient.** In general, I think people can eat anything they damn well please – **in reason and tempered.** The body knows how to throw away what it doesn't want, what it doesn't need, what it doesn't recognize. However, if you are bombarding it with SAD (the Standard American Diet), the body will accumulate a buildup, and a buildup is a disorder or disease.

There are optimal ways to approach food that will help your system work more smoothly and stay healthier. We'll look at the components of a "Stay Healthy Diet" in Chapter 8.

Being Slim – A Numbers Game

More and more scary information is coming out daily linking extra pounds with developing some serious health issues. When you weigh too much, you're at a higher risk for everything from heart disease, to high blood pressure, to diabetes, to even some cancers. There are so many diet options out there that it gets confusing. So let's boil it all down to basic weight-loss secrets that you need to know.

Here's the first secret: especially us girls as we get older, we've got to remember that being at the right weight is a numbers game. And the numbers are this; on average, if a person eats 2200 calories a day, their weight will stay exactly where it is. But if you eat 500 EXTRA calories every day for a week (2200 + 500 extra = 2700 calories daily), you will gain one pound by Day 7. That's because 3500 extra calories (7 days x 500 extra calories a day) equals one pound of weight gain.

So if you're noticing that the pounds have been coming on, you need to ask yourself if you were stressing … did someone did someone at work piss you off? What was the deal? Because usually when we eat too much, the deal is *stress*. It might be a divorce … fighting for custody of a child or even a pet … maybe a parent has passed away. And you started eating more than usual… and it was junk food, fast food, salty food, fried food, sugar, etc. The event was a cue you needed to start smothering your feelings or block them out with food.

So you started racking up the calories. Soon you were feeling miserable. But it didn't happen overnight. You gained the weight over time. Then you woke up and wondered, "How did I get here?" I often ask my clients, "At what point did you recognize that you had a problem?" or "When did you recognize that you were in trouble?" At least, at some point, these clients woke up and came to see me. However, in other cases, the person doesn't snap back into reality. Some people just want to feel better, so they continue to eat more than they need. How about you? Are you still in denial about a weight issue?

Remember, it's a numbers game. Here is the next set of numbers … *If you want to lose weight, what you need to do calorie-wise is eat less than the 2200 calories – let's say 1900 calories. Then go out there and burn off another 300-400 calories or more a day through exercise.*

THE STANDARD AMERICAN DIET (SAD)

It used to be when we were younger that we could eat just about anything and we wouldn't gain weight. *Not kids today.* These days, the children gain weight because they're eating junk. Fast foods are not created to be health food! Plus kids are not moving enough … they're sitting in front of the TV or the computer too many hours of the day.

When your lifestyle dictates that you are eating at the fast food places for breakfast, lunch and dinner, your diet is going to be out of balance, and your body will get sick. These high-fat, high-sodium (salt), low-nutrition meals were not designed for how many calories you need. One meal from a fast food restaurant can contain most of the calories your body requires for the entire day. *One meal!* And people are doing this all the time! Because it's convenient. Because it's there. It tastes good. And the food manufacturers design it with ingredients that will keep you coming back for more of the same stuff. So for three days in a row, you may have the same fast food sandwich with fries or chips.

True Story: Get Real

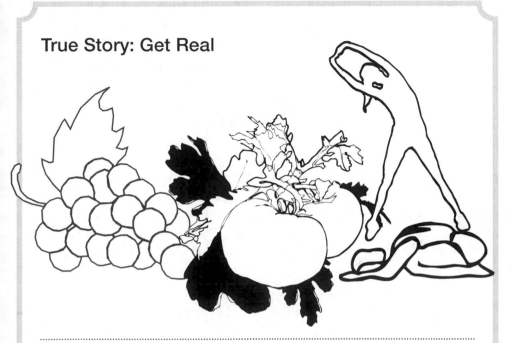

I had a client who worked out like a banshee, every day, at the age of 43. She was working out like a dog, but ate like a horse. Unfortunately, she had a craving for sugar and a junk food habit. I said to her, "You're eating more than you're burning up through your exercise. That's why the pounds aren't coming off." People have to be realistic.

Here's a weight loss secret to add to the numbers game idea: **if you want to lose or maintain weight, you've got to become aware of what racks up the calories.** Many times, it's junk foods. Also ... here comes another secret: **learn how many calories are in the nutritious foods you want to eat, and make those better choices.** If you know that six strawberries are 24 calories (about 4 each), an orange is 65 calories, and a banana is (depends on how green or yellow and spotty it is) about 100-110 calories, you can keep your caloric intake down, and eat good nutritious foods all day long. Then just take a walk or two a day to get to or to maintain the desired weight.

Plus, you chase it down with soda. You order a greasy burger, and eat it with an ice-cold soda. You don't even half-chew the burger. Then you swallow it with the chilled soda, which solidifies the grease. So now you've got little chunks of the hard fat going through your system. How nasty is that?

Read this for a real eye-opener:

LUNCH AT MCDONALD'S
(Figures from www.mcdonalds.com.)

Double Quarter Pounder with Cheese®
740 calories / 19 gm saturated fat / 1380 mg sodium

Chocolate Triple Thick® Shake (16 fl oz)
580 calories / 8 gm saturated fat / 250 mg sodium

French Fries (medium size)
380 calories / 2.5 gm saturated fat / 270 mg sodium

Total
1700 calories / 29.5 gm saturated fat / 1900 mg sodium

At 2200 calories a day, you'd have only 500 calories left for the rest of your food! And look at the sodium! The American Heart Association recommends you consume no more than 2400 mg of sodium a day. You're getting close to the AHA's

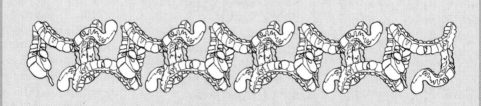

CONSIDER THESE STATS & FACTS

According to the Centers for Disease Control, an alarming **one in three** Americans was considered obese in 2006-2007.

Over the last three decades, the rate of obesity **has tripled** in the US.

Blacks have the highest rates of obesity (45%), followed by Mexican-Americans (37%).

Obesity is associated with more ill health, reduced quality of life, and a higher risk for premature death, reports the CDC.

Making healthier food choices, reducing portion sizes, and becoming more physically active were among the top approaches the CDC recommends for fighting obesity.

The CDC agrees that having a healthy weight isn't just about a "diet" or "program." It's part of an ongoing healthier lifestyle.

limit with this one meal. And at this same level of calories, the AHA says to eat no more than 18 grams of saturated fat. This meal goes way beyond that. Add a slice of Marie Calendar's apple pie (570 calories) and an 8-ounce glass of whole milk (150 calories), and you'd be more than done for the day.

How about trying a tuna sandwich for lunch at Subway? Sounds healthy …

LUNCH AT SUBWAY

(Figures from http://www.subway.com/ and http://www.pepsiproductfacts.com/.)

6" Tuna Sandwich

530 calories / 6 gm saturated fat / 950 mg sodium

Lays Classic Potato Chips – Snack Size

230 calories / 2 gm saturated fat / 270 mg sodium

Pepsi (21 oz)

262 calories / 0 gm saturated fat / 52 mg sodium

Total

1022 calories / 7.5 gm saturated fat / 1272 mg sodium

Is this a healthy meal? No, not so much. The calories and sodium in the fish sub are about as high as in a Big Mac (540 calories/1040 mg sodium) at McDonald's. It's amazing!

Check out your favorite McDonald's and Subway meals at the sites listed above. You'll be surprised by what you find.

Here's something I found so troubling. A friend was telling me that she had to eat on the run one day several years ago, so she ate at McDonald's – not her usual routine. There was a mother and daughter in front of her in line, and they both were in a McDonald's contest where you got a credit for every time you ate there. Once you reached a certain level, McDonald's would give you a bonus. To me, that is so SAD. As you can see from the example above, a McDonald's habit wouldn't be healthy for the mother or the daughter, but they were reinforcing each other's behavior.

This past July, McDonald's reported a 4.3% increase in same-store sales, reportedly due to pressure people are feeling from the economy. Folks, if you're eating fast food 'cause you're watching your pennies, know that there are healthier ways to eat for less money. Even if you tell yourself that you're going to be buying healthier choices there, you can still find more nutritious food someplace else that isn't costly.

My answer is simple when a client tells me that they eat a lot of fast food. I just tell them that they're off of it. And I say, "All I am asking is that you give me two, or three, or four days, and see how much better you feel. See how much this helps your system." And most of them will do it. They go off it completely. And they do feel better.

WHAT'S YOUR THING?

Sugar Cravings

One of the biggest issues that I see for women is **sugar**. From the digestion perspective, think about this. Sugar is sticky, it's gooey. When heat hits it (like in your digestive tract), it gets tacky.

Not so good for smooth moves in the bathroom.

Sugar can overload your adrenal glands (which help govern your stress level). One of the worst things about sugar is that it is at the top of the list of foods that can make your system acidic.

Stress throughout the day makes us want to have sugar. But know this: too much sugar throws the whole body's balance off. It strips your body of its natural intelligence. You think you're doing something normal, but you're doing something crazy. And it's the sugar doing it.

There's a story that I like to share with my clients, because I remember going through it myself years ago. And when I tell it to people, they nod their head in acknowledgement the whole time.

You're on your way home from work. You say to yourself, "I don't have any sugar at my house. I'm going straight home. I'm not going to stop at the Seven 11 to get a candy bar."

You keep saying to yourself, "I'm not going to do it. I'm not going to do it." But before you know it, you're turning into the Seven 11 parking lot.

And you say to yourself with reason, "I'm not going to buy any candy. I'm just going to get a bottled water. And I'm coming out of there." Soon you're headed back to your car, and you've got six candy bars and a bottle of water!

Now you say to yourself, "I'm just going to have a little piece to take the edge off." But then you eat that whole candy bar and start the second one.

This kind of crazy behavior comes from sugar addiction. Yes, sugar is a drug. When you eat sugar, your body starts telling you, "I want more, and more, and more." It's like cigarettes, or cocaine, or any other kind of addiction. It will rob from your body, steal and destroy.

If people tell me that they are a sugar junky, I ask, "What kind of sugar do you crave? Do you crave the hard stuff, like chocolate bars? The hard candy? Do you crave the donuts and the cakes? What is it?" It's important to be aware of what you're doing. That way, you can make changes.

There's the sugar made from low-grade refined cane sugar and then there is the high fructose sweeteners. Both cause an instant spiking of the glycemic rate. In contrast, a natural unrefined sweetener like agave nectar has a lower glycemic load.

I'll say to my sugar-craving client, "Do me a favor. Give me three days without eating sugar. Because I know that you can do this. You're an intelligent individual. Stop eating any sugar for three days. And I guarantee you that you'll, first of all, lose weight. That's number 1. And number 2, you're going to feel so much better at the end of it. Initially, it may seem like you can't do it because you're hooked on sugar. However, if you stick with it, this will become easy to do for three days. If you can do it for three days, you can do it for four; all I'm asking for is three days."

I want them to know that they can do it.

Because right then, when I'm talking to them, it can feel like they can't.

If you're going off sugar, know that you're likely to be mean, cantankerous, and a tad bit on the evil side. But this phase will pass.

Now there are some people who are going to need support from supplements to get over their sugar addiction. There's a combination of supplements that I've seen to be very helpful. The main supplement is L-Glutamine, which is an amino acid. It's great for helping to balance the body's sugar level. Glutamine is also a major fuel source for our bodies.

The other supplements are the fatty acid Alpha-Lipoic Acid (ALA), the mineral Chromium, and the amino acid 5-HTP. The 5-HTP helps facilitate the effectiveness of the other supplements in this group. I also add vitamin B-complex capsules.

The dosage is:
- two 500-mg capsules of L-Glutamine twice a day
- two 250-mg capsules of Alpha Lopoic Acid twice a day
- one 200-mg Chromium once a day
- one capsule 5-HTP once a day
- two B-complex capsules once a day (mornings only)

So when you're craving sugar and you're serious about getting off of it, this is the combination to use. You take it at this level for one week or however long it takes for you to get over your sugar cravings. Everyone's system is different.

If you're still stressing for a while, you can add the amino acid DL Phenylalanine, Coenzyme Q10 (Co-Q10) and a good Liquid Multi-Nutrient (such as intraMax [available through Drucker Labs via my website]). These supplements can help you achieve a sense of well-being.

The additions to the combination are:
- two 500-mg capsules of DL Phenylalanine three times a day for the 1st week (Reduce to 2 capsules a day the 2nd week.)
- one 60-mg Co-Q10 once a day
- daily dose of a Liquid Multi-Nutrient

A good book for sugar junkies to read is *The Diet Cure* by Julia Ross. It explains how to overcome chemical imbalances in the body. Another one is *Sugar Blues* by William Dufty.

Of course, check with your doctor before starting any new vitamin regimen.

There's one other problem with sugar that I want to bring to your attention. Sugar feeds the yeast in your body. Everybody has yeast in their body; we're born with it. You may have heard it referred to as Candida, which is the Latin word for yeast. Candida resides naturally in our digestive tract.

If you feed the yeast sugar, it's going to love it. And it's going to overgrow.

Have you ever started itching after eating a candy bar? You have a feeding frenzy going on. One thing that you want to avoid is a yeast problem. You don't want to get the yeast in your body all flared up and out of control. See the supplement chapter for information on a 90-Day Candida Control Program.

Loving the Carbs

Then I have the people who say, "Oh no, I don't eat a lot of sugar. I don't eat a lot of sweets." So I ask them, "What about your **carbs**? What is your carb intake like?" And they'll say, "On my God, I love the carbs." They're falling out thinking about it. And I'll reply, "OK, that's your sugar. For the next three days, no carbs." And they do it! Yet their first thought was "there's nothing else to eat." So I instantly point out the things that they can have. And that they *will* get full, and they'll be OK. They're not going to pass out and die from not eating carbs.

I tell them that they can eat all the fish, chicken and turkey that they like. And fresh vegetables. And all the salads in the world. Just stay away from carbs – bread, pasta, cookies, etc. And if you fall off the wagon, you decide that you have to have a carb today, during that three days, then make sure that you do not eat it with any of the protein. So then I'm getting them used to food combining.

Since they feel better by eating just the way I've described, they tend to stick with it. When I see them after the two to four days of them doing exactly what I said, and maybe they've gone out or something, but they still are on it for the most part, they notice that their acid reflux has gone away. Or it's not as bad. And by the time they come in to see me, they feel like I've created a miracle. And they want that feeling to last. Because most people don't know how bad they feel until they start to feel good. And food can really make you feel bad. Most people want to feel better.

If someone wants to feel bad, then they've accepted feeling miserable, and I can't help those people. And I tell them that. I ask, "Why are you coming to me? You can be sick and die all by yourself. I don't need to participate in this nonsense."

What's your choice? Are you willing to make some changes or do you accept feeling miserable?

The Soda Habit

I've found that people who love sodas lose track of how much they're drinking (and how much of it is flowing through their system). It used to be that a cola would come in an 6- or 8-ounce bottle. Now we've got the Big Gulp (32 oz), the Super Big Gulp (41 or 44 oz), and the Double Gulp (64 oz) at the convenience stores. Whenever you over-consume soda, your liver has to work overtime. The average American drinks one gallon (128 oz) of soda a week.

Right now, there's a big story in India about how farmers are spraying their fields with Coke to keep their crops free of bugs. An Indian watchdog group, the Centre for Science and the Environment, released a report earlier that the drink purportedly has high levels of pesticide residues. While the source of the pesticides is thought to perhaps be the local water, who knows? Whatever the truth is in India, Americans are ingesting pesticides from some items in their food – most likely from fruit, vegetables and dairy. A 2009 Centers for Disease Control study found pesticides in blood and urine samples of nearly 96% of the more than 5,000 Americans it tested. Another CDC-affiliated study found pesticide residues in mother's milk from all 400 women tested.

I've long thought of soda as poison, and one of the known offending ingredients is high-fructose corn syrup. Also, many people drink diet-sodas all day long, without a thought about the dangerous artificial sweeteners they're consuming. If you think you're off the hook with sugar-sweetened soft drinks, know that they're strongly associated with weight gain, diabetes, and dental cavities. To top it off, the Center for Science in the Public Interest identified nutritional depletion among soda drinkers, in a report that found soda consumption to be soaring, particularly among children.

When a new client tells me they drink soda, I suggest that they try cutting it out of their diet entirely for one month. It takes 30 days to make or break a habit, so I ask them to give it a solid month. Most of these people don't want to go back to the sodas after that time. I recommend that they have water as their drink of choice. And I say that they can add lemon and a little juice to give the water some flavor.

People find that they begin to lose unwanted pounds, with just this one change. They are also reducing their risk of diabetes, high blood pressure and heart disease.

Over-Doing the Meat Habit

I am finding overeating meat to be a major issue, especially among men. From what I've observed, it seems that the black man eats more red meat than any other humans on this planet. An adult black male will leave work, stop to have a hamburger or hot dog along the way, and then go home and have a steak for dinner.

Here are the issues with meat. First of all, animal protein is harder to digest than the other foods. If you're overeating meat, it's going to create havoc in the system – especially when combined with the wrong foods. Your body is going to back up, and you'll have a hard time eliminating. And when that meat is stored in your system, it is going to putrefy. (Got Gout?)

Also, according to WebMD, many studies have shown that "people who eat the most meat get the most cancer." And a study from the American Cancer Society took an even closer look. They found that those who eat the most red meat, including beef and pork, get colon cancer 30-40% more often than people who just eat these foods occasionally. A study spokeswoman suggests that it is best to think of red meat as a special treat, not a daily food item.

Research has also found that fresh meats are better than processed meats (hot dogs, sausage and cold cuts). Chemicals added in processing the meat add to your cancer risk.

A 10-year observational study funded by the National Cancer Institute provides some hard numbers for what is too much. Those with the higher risk diets ate 62.5 grams of meat a day on average, seven times that of the lowest risk group.

You want to avoid eating that much meat, no matter how much you like it. If your belly is expanding, chances are that you are wearing that cow. And the Guernsey is going to take you down, just like you took it down. That is, if you're not careful with your meat consumption.

The Mayo Clinic recommends only eating about 3-ounces of meat a day, which is about the size of a deck of cards. I personally think that is too much, especially with the consumption of foods like pizza, breads, other carbs and no veggies. Eating too much meat increases your risk of colon cancer, other cancers such as prostate cancer, heart disease, and death. Eating less meat is easier if you don't think of the meat as the focus of your meal. If you still crave your red meat, cut it back to at least once a month.

Bottom line: You want to eat meat in a manner that allows the body to move it through your system in a healthy way. If you've been overdoing it and need to clear out your system, try Dr. Schulze's herbal formula called the Bowel Flush Shot. When people come to see me and they need this step, I suggest that they take one of these shots each day for three days. The shots come in a pack of three.

If you crave protein, make it a lighter one such as fish, chicken or turkey. Look for kosher or free-range chicken and turkey, and wild caught fish to avoid toxins and chemicals.

FOOD COMBINING BASICS
Earlier in this chapter, I mentioned "food combining." Let's look at the proper food-combining principles.

When you eat your protein, you should eat it with vegetables only. That is an excellent combination. When you eat your carbohydrates, you should eat them with vegetables only. Another excellent combination. But what you don't want to do is combine your proteins and your carbs together.

When you eat animal protein, it takes an acid enzyme to break it down. When you eat a carbohydrate, it takes an alkaline enzyme to break it down. You might remember the following from high school: when you put two chemicals, one acid and one alkaline, together, they neutralize each other. Therefore if you mix proteins and carbs, you won't digest your food well. So you're going to end up with rotting meat moving through your gut, and partially digested carbs, which are sugar, moving through a hot canal and fermenting! Because that's what sugar does when it gets into heat like that. It tends to ferment. So now you've got gas.

If you have been wondering why you've been so gassy lately, that could be one of the reasons.

To avoid this, eat your protein with vegetables only, and eat your carbs with vegetables only. And if you slip up, you want to get the supplement **Activated Charcoal** which will get rid of the gas and move it right through your system. Activated Charcoal is what they give you in a hospital when you have food poisoning. It just pulls out the poisons, like the gas. You take 1 teaspoon mixed in water or juice once a day for no more than one week. Sometimes the directions will say to take a capful or it may come in capsules. In those cases, read the directions.

Bottoms Up! (What to Drink)

Water should be your drink of choice. *Always*. As I've mentioned in the colonics chapter, you want to be drinking half of your body weight in ounces daily. Why? Well, every single cell in your body needs water in order to function and to live. Drinking water is one way we can take good care of ourselves and our cells.

If you drink **juices**, you want natural juices – not processed juices with added corn syrup or artificial ingredients like chemical coloring agents. You can juice it on your own, or you'll want to dilute your commercial all-natural juice with water, and then squeeze lemon in it. This drink will taste like slightly sweetened lemonade. And since you've watered it down, your body won't have to fight it to get rid of the sugar.

If you're going to be drinking alcohol, your alcoholic beverage should be **red wine only**. But not the cheap wines that have been sweetened up. Instead, drink the Merlots, the Sauvignons, the Burgundies. And that is the only beverage that I recommend you drink with a meal. Not even water should be drunk with a meal. But red wine is OK because you don't drink it, you sip it. Secondly, it gives the appearance to the body that it's food coming down. Because red wine has antioxidants in it ... to help with the blood. And it has enzymes in it to help with digestion.

Instead of at mealtime, drink your water at least a half hour before or 45 minutes after a meal. If you're chewing your foods well, you won't have to be drinking anything with a meal anyway! Most people drink to help wash the food down. They should be chewing their food better.

Let's not forget to think about how to handle **coffee**. Obviously, it's very popular; eight out of 10 Americans drink it every day. Just look at how many Starbucks there are. Despite its popularity, there are reasons to be concerned about coffee. One of the problems is that it's quite addictive, mostly because of the caffeine. Also, it over-stimulates the body. In addition, coffee has been shown to cause cell mutations, and it's been linked with bladder and breast cancer. If you have to have your coffee, keep it to just one cup a day. Keep in mind that for each cup of coffee that you drink, it strips the body of about seven glasses of water. In other words, coffee is very dehydrating for your body.

An alternative to coffee that I drink and recommend to my clients is organic Rooibos – "rooi" means "red" and "bos" means "bush" – herbal tea from African Red Tea Imports. It is naturally caffeine-free, high in antioxidants, and rich in minerals such as selenium. Unlike a light herbal tea like chamomile, Rooibos creates a dark tea when you brew it. Harvested from a mountain slope near Cape Town in South Africa, this is a very nutritious type of red tea which has long been treasured as an elixir for the mind, body and spirit. The tea is available in bags, loose and as a powder (which is its most antioxidant-rich form for anti-aging). It comes in a variety of combinations, such as a blend with vanilla bean or African ginger. Learn more at www.africanredtea.com.

Steer Clear of Fried Foods

Generally, I tell my clients that they should not eat anything fried, unless it is fried in olive oil. That is about the only oil that I usually recommend anyway. Coconut oil is fine, too.

It's actually a good idea to steer clear of fried food totally. Why? Well, most processed oil is already tainted before you even open up the bottle or can. But you can't tell that it's rancid. The problem is that oil doesn't stay fresh very long. And we can't tell how long that oil has been sitting on the shelf. What happens is that they process the oil, and then it sits on the shelf until you buy it. And that's like buying packaged baked goods, rather than going to a bakery where they make the food fresh every day.

So now you have rancid oil, with a rancidity that you can't smell because of the processing. However, the body knows that it's gone bad. It's very smart.

People buy their oil. It looks clear. It smells fine. But the minute you heat it up to a certain temperature, it changes the molecular structure of the oil. So now, as an example, let's say that it goes from being an O molecule to an X molecule. And the X molecule is like that sticky yellowish stuff that you see on the wall of a kitchen where they've done a lot of deep frying. That stuff is tough to

get off. Try spraying a little Mr. Clean on it. That is a joke. Then you take a spatula and try to scrap it off. It's not happening. It's doing the same thing in your arteries. That's a serious buildup.

Now people will say to me, "Well, I only eat fried fish once a week. Every Friday." And I tell them, "Those Fridays add up. There's one Friday, then the next one, then the next one, then the next one. Plus, it's not just the fried foods that you're eating that are causing the problem. If we added those other things into it, we can honestly say that eventually your body is going to catch up with you. Even though blood may be pumping fully through your arteries right now."

They call it "plaque," and it makes the arteries stiff and narrow from the fat that has thickened, like the oil on the kitchen walls. And when the arteries are stiff and less wide, that means the heart has to pump harder. That means your blood pressure will be up. And this is what happens.

So fried food … I say not.

Olive oil in a salad, OK. But get it from a reliable source. If you're getting it from a cheap bargain store, think again.

Go Organic

I recommend organic for everything. If it's not organic, green or natural, I stay away from it. I do go out to dinner and go to parties where the food is not organic. However, I don't overdo it and I know when to back off. I know what's not good for me. The most important thing is that I go organic most of the time.

We know very little about the long-term effects of ingesting pesticide residues. According to the Environmental Working Group, one effect that has been found is increased neurological problems in children. Governmental agencies, like the state of California, are working to reduce pesticide use. However, their progress is slow. The power to reduce your exposure to pesticides is in how you spend your shopping dollars. Whenever you can, go organic.

A study published in *Environmental Health Perspectives* showed that the signs of eating organic show up fairly quickly. Children who had biological markers of pesticides in their urine later had no signs after switching to organic fruits, vegetables and juices. In addition to looking for organic produce, one of the study authors, Chensheng Li, had an additional suggestion. He recommended buying produce from local farmers you know who minimize their use of pesticides. You can get to know the produce growers at your local farmers markets.

Don't Forget Your Fiber

Well, I can't write a nutrition chapter as a colon hydrotherapist without addressing fiber. First, there are two types of fiber – *soluble* and *insoluble.* And you can do too much of one or the other. If you eat too much insoluble fiber, you make it difficult for the small intestines to absorb the nutrients from your food. (I see this mostly in my raw food clients who are eating too much coarse fiber.) If you do too much of the soluble fiber,

what you're going to have is a blockage. You'll be totally constipated.

What soluble fiber does is it bulks up once the moisture hits it. Insoluble fiber sweeps right on through. It doesn't bulk as a rule. It just moves food along. Many people just do soluble fiber and think they're getting enough fiber. Well, they're not. When you have a good combination of the two types of fiber, you'll have better digestion.

By the way, the commercial fiber product Benefiber, as far as I am considered, is the worse commercial stuff on the planet. I say this because I have unclogged so many people after they took Benefiber.

On their website, they tell you that you can take Benefiber Powder "any way you choose." (However, carbonated beverages are not recommended.) So you can put it in your coffee, in your water, in your juice. And then you drink it. People are doing this every day when they don't even need that much fiber. And they think it's good because the doctor told them, "Get a little more fiber in your diet."

Sources of soluble fiber include: oatmeal; dried legumes such as lima beans, black eyed peas and lentils; some fruits like apples, bananas, peaches and pears; and certain vegetable such as broccoli, Brussels sprouts and carrots. Sources of insoluble fiber are whole grain foods like breads; nuts and seeds; and vegetables such as green beans, celery and cauliflower.

You'll want to eat between 25 and 40 grams of fiber each day. In general,

True Story
Watch Out for the Commercial Fiber Products

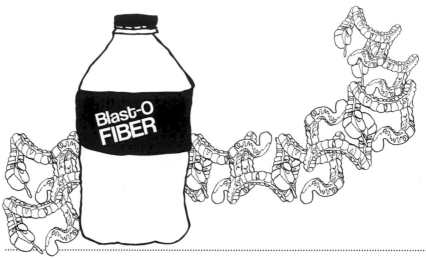

In one case, it took me a whole week to unclog a client after she took Benefiber. She was a beautiful older woman who got into that kind of trouble, and she sought me out. She had been taking Benefiber in her coffee every day. Coffee constipates anyway; it dries the body up. This woman noticed that she went from having great bowel movements, to OK bowel movements, to no bowel movement. When she came to me, she hadn't pooped in a week. This beautiful lady was just beside herself!

When I talked to her over the phone, she trusted that I would do the job. I warned her that it wasn't going to happen overnight. And we did a colonic every day because she had plans to go out of town. Finally I sent her to Dr. Schulze for his Intestinal Formula One, and this did the trick working from the top down. (I had been working from the bottom out.) And when it finally broke through, it was like heaven. But this wasn't until Friday night, and this client was leaving the next day for her trip to visit with friends in New York City. She did still go to one more appointment with another colon hydrotherapist who I recommend in New York and she was able to have a good time with her girlfriends in the Big Apple.

according to Columbia University, Americans barely take in about 50% of the fiber they need each day.

Remember, meat has zero fiber.

What about Dairy?

Yes, dairy has calcium in it, but you can get calcium from spinach and other dark leafy vegetables. As far as I am concerned, I'd rather do supplements than do the dairy foods. Eighty percent of the entire planet is lactose intolerant anyway. But big business has us believing that dairy is good for the body.

To me, milk is liquid *from another animal*. It's like drinking the cow's blood. And it can be constipating; however, for those who are lactose intolerant, milk can trigger diarrhea.

There's the ad that asks, "Got Milk?" I say, "Not milk."

If you're going to eat cheese, I recommend "doing the real thing." Avoid what they call "government cheese" ("gov'ment cheese") or processed cheese. Those will constipate you for sure. Do the white cheese, not cheese with food coloring and other additives in it like chemical preservatives, artificial flavors, and flavor enhancers such as monosodium glutamate or yeast extract. And don't eat too much of the cheese.

I like soy cheese, which is made from soymilk. There's a white Pepper Jack Soy Cheese I buy that's really very good. And since it melts like real cheese, you can make mac and cheese with it.

Bottom line, you have to be careful and make good choices when it comes to dairy. Plus, you want to go back to the idea of "too much is unnecessary and too little is inefficient." You don't want to ever overdo it. There are people out there who eat cheese just like it is candy. Then they wonder why their system is clogged up and their skin is bad.

The Zero Years

I recommend that you reassess how you're eating every 10 years because the body's needs change over time. I call these turning points "the zero years" – ages 10, 20, 30, 40, 50, 60, etc. The changes can be devastating if you don't pay attention. And it's all based around your body's needs and wants.

For example, in the teen years, you might get away with eating lots of non-nutritious foods like pizza or peanut butter and jelly sandwiches. However, in your 20s, your body starts going through biological changes. You start feeling the effects of too much pizza. If you don't change your diet by the time you turn 30, it's going to really hit you then. Certain nutrients are no longer produced by the body. Your hair starts to change, and your skin begins to show signs of aging. The digestive tract changes too. You may notice that your belly bloats each time you eat. Maybe you realize that you need to ease up a bit. And the years march on.

By the time you're 50, you may find yourself staring in the mirror at a person you don't recognize.

Too many people in their mid-30s feel and look like they're in their 40s or 50s. Wouldn't you rather eat and live smart, and look and feel 30 at 40, and 40 at 50?

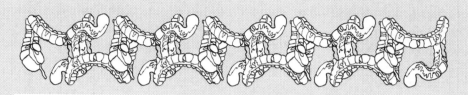

EATING FOR GOOD DIGESTION

1. Chew, chew, chew your food well.

2. Don't eat and drink at the same time. (Occasionally a little red wine is OK.)

3. Don't combine your proteins and your carbs.

4. Don't stuff yourself; follow the 80/20 rule. Eat until you feel 80% full, then stop. The reason? It takes your brain 20 minutes to catch up with the fact that you're full. If you keep eating, you'll overdo it.

5. Remember to get your share of fiber (25 to 40 grams a day).

Balance Your Diet
Alkaline & Acid Foods

When your body metabolizes food, the end products will turn out to be either alkaline or acid. The charts below show the foods that are Alkaline Forming and Acid Forming. Your body strives to keep itself in balance. When the internal body is too acidic, it becomes a breeding ground for disease. It is more vulnerable to infectious microorganisms. You will also feel out of whack. The Standard American Diet is highly acidic.

You'll want to eat foods from both sides of the chart on the following page. The ratio to aim for is about 80% alkaline and 20% acidic.

Note: Agave nectar is only slightly acidic. In comparison, artificial sweeteners are very acidic. The thing I like about agave nectar is that it is a low glycemic index food, meaning that its sugar is absorbed by the body at a slower rate than sugar or honey.

Your Turn

Since we can't see on the inside, we don't know exactly what shape our body is in. We don't know what we're doing to ourselves when we drink too much coffee, eat too much meat, overdo the sugar, etc. When we do these things, and we don't "get it" yet, we are killing ourselves consistently.

A lot of times all we need to do is cut back, cut down, and cut out certain things, and the body will start rejuvenating itself ... renewing itself! This chapter has given you direction for where you want to be headed. Now it's your turn to choose to start eating better!

Alkaline & Acid Foods

80% ALKALINE FORMING FOODS

VEGETABLES
Alfalfa
Asparagus
Barley grass
Beets
Broccoli
Brussels sprouts
Cabbage
Carrot
Cauliflower
Celery
Chard
Chlorella
Collard greens
Cucumber
Dandelions
Dulce
Edible flowers
Eggplant
Fermented veggies
Garlic
Kale
Kohlrabi
Lettuce
Mushrooms
Mustard greens
Nightshade veggies
Onions
Parsnips (high gly)
Peas
Peppers
Pumpkin
Rutabaga
Sea veggies
Spirulina
Sprouts
Squashes
Watercress
Wheat grass
Wild greens

FRUITS
Apple
Apricot
Avocado
Banana (high gly)
Berries
Cantaloupe
Cherries
Currants
Dates/figs
Grapefruit
Grapes
Honeydew melon
Lemon
Lime
Nectarine
Orange
Peach
Pear
Pineapple
Tangerines
Tomato
Tropical fruits
Watermelon

PROTEIN
Almonds
Chestnuts
Chicken breast
Cottage cheese
Eggs (poached)
Flax seeds
Millet
Pumpkin seeds
Sprouted seeds
Squash seeds
Sunflower seeds
Tempeh (fermented)
Tofu (fermented)
Whey powder
Yogurt

OTHER
Alkaline antioxidant
Apple cider vinegar
Banchi tea
Bee pollen
Dandelion tea
Fresh fruit juice
Ginseng tea
Green juices
Green tea
Herbal tea
Kombucha
Lecithin granules
Mineral water
Organic milk
(unpasteurized)
Probiotic cultures
Veggie juices

SWEETENER
Stevia

SPICES/SEASONINGS
All herbs
Chili pepper
Cinnamon
Curry
Ginger
Miso
Mustard
Sea salt
Tamari

ORIENTAL VEGGIES
Daikon
Dandelion root
Kombu
Maitake
Nori
Reishi
Sea veggies
Shitake
Umeboshi
Wakame

20% ACID FORMING FOODS

FATS & OILS
Avocado oil
Canola oil
Corn oil
Hemp seed oil
Flax oil
Lard
Olive oil
Safflower oil
Sesame oil
Sunflower oil

FRUITS
Cranberries

GRAINS
Amaranth
Barley
Buckwheat
Corn
Hemp seed flour
Kamut
Oats (rolled)
Quinoa
Rice (all)
Rice cakes
Rye
Spelt
Wheat
Wheat cakes

NUTS
Almond milk
Brazil nuts
Cashews
Peanut butter
Peanuts
Pecans
Tahini
Walnuts

ANIMAL PROTEIN
Carp
Clams
Fish
Lamb
Lobster
Mussels
Oysters
Rabbit
Salmon
Scallops
Tuna
Turkey
Venison

OTHER
Distilled vinegar
Potatoes
Wheat germ
Agave nectar
Honey

COMPOUNDS
Aspartame

CHEMICALS
Drugs, Medicinal
Drugs, Psychedelic
Herbicides
Pesticides

ALCOHOL
Beer
Hard Liquor
Spirits
Wine

BEANS & LEGUMES
Black beans
Chick peas
Green beans
Kidney beans
Lentils
Lima beans
Pinto beans
Red beans
Rice milk
Soy beans
Soy milk
White beans

Remember, *too much is unnecessary, and too little is inefficient.* The body is looking for balance, aka homeostasis, all of the time. If you eat in a balanced way, your body will do its job. And it will fight to do its job, by sending you signals when you go off track. For example, I have observed that most people who go off red meat for a couple months feel sicker than a dog when they try to go back to it. Their body is protesting because it has been allowed to become balanced with the good food the person has been taking in. When the person throws that monkey wrench into the works, the body completely goes into a tailspin.

Many diseases are asymptomatic (display no early symptoms). By the time they really show up, it can be too late. Do things now – like improving your diet – that can keep those bad boys out of the picture of your life.

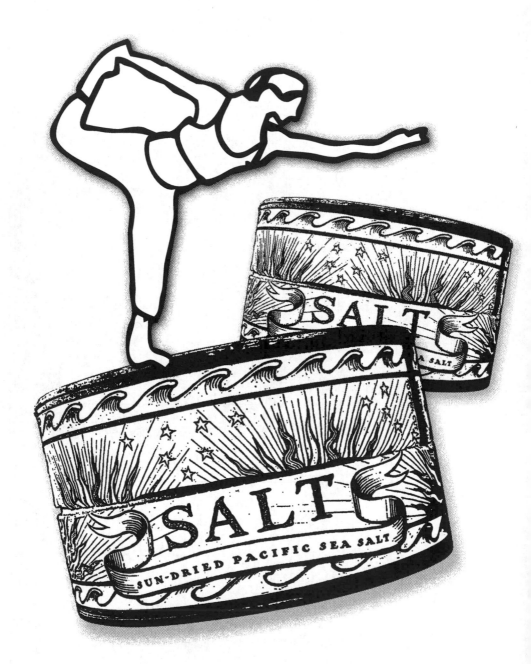

CHAPTER 9

Blood, Sweat & Tears

The human blood contains 0.9% salt (sodium chloride). Sodium (salt) is essential for life.

Sodium comes in many forms. You may have heard the different forms referred to by the following names: sodium phosphate, sodium acetate, sodium bicarbonate and sodium chloride.

In the human body, sodium works in conjunction with potassium for a balanced effect on blood pressure. According to an article in **Whole Foods** magazine, a good way to consume enough potassium is to eat natural, unprocessed foods.

Meanwhile, sodium and chloride are both electrolytes. They conduct electricity through water and allow electrical nerve impulses to pass from cell to cell. A body without electrolytes will collapse.

Have you ever noticed just how salty we are?

BLOOD IS SALTY.
SWEAT IS SALTY.
TEARS ARE SALTY.
PEE IS SALTY.

These fluid substances contain an average of 0.9% parts of dissolved salt. The human body is 70-80% water and .9% of that is salt. How amazing is it that over 70% of the earth is covered by oceans, and that water is 3.5% salt.

Human life cannot exist without salt. It maintains the electrolyte balance inside and outside cells. When your doctor does a routine physical examination. she or he will measure electrolytes for clues of personal health.

Sodium, chloride and potassium can be affected by several medicines. Abnormalities can cause an abnormal heartbeat, as an example. Inadequate amounts of salt can be problematic. Doctors often recommend replacing water and salt lost in exercise to maintain hydration when working out.

Believe it or not, increased salt intake has been used successfully to combat Chronic Fatigue Syndrome. (Always check with your physician before starting new measures of health remedies.)

Most of our salt comes from foods, some from water. Our regular table-salt no longer has anything in common with the original crystal salt. The problem with salt is not the salt itself but the condition of the salt we eat! Sodium chloride is not what the body recognizes.

With the advent of industrial development, our natural salt was "chemically cleaned" and reduced only to sodium and chloride (low-grade table salt). It is essentially poisoned. In contrast, sea salt or rock salt is like medicine.

Sodium chloride has adverse effects on the human body. The common table-salt we use for cooking has only two or three chemical elements.

Seawater has 84 chemical elements. It is essential for the human body to have at least 60 of these minerals in order to maintain a disease-free and ailment-free state.

BRIME

I have found that a mixture of Karisalt brime (made with Karisalt Andes Pink [Sea] Salt) and Kangen alkaline water (7.0 pH) taken every morning can harmonize the alkaline balance in the body and normalize blood pressure.

Karisalt's Andes Pink Salt is by far the best salt. This pink mineral salt was formed over three hundred million years ago. A pure deep ocean evaporated, and the salt was buried under the Andes Mountains, which protected this reserve from pollutants. The incredible weight of the mountains over long periods of time transformed the salt into a very special form of crystallized rock salt. Andes pink salt has no sediment, and it is not refined. It is mined, crushed and delivered in a natural state.

PREPARATION OF KARISALT (BRIME) WATER

1. Put several Andes pink salt rocks in a closable 10-ounce glass container. Add Kangen 7.0 water, and completely fill the container.
2. Let it sit for at least 24 hours, then check and see if the pink salt rocks have completely dissolved. If so, add a few more pink salt rocks to the solution. When the pink salt rocks can no longer be dissolved, the solution has finally become saturated at 26% and is ready to drink. The 26% concentration of the solution remains stable.

3. Put a teaspoon of this Brime in a 8.5-ounce glass of Kangen water and drink it on a empty stomach every morning. Wait at least 20 minutes before eating or drinking anything else.
4. You can refill the glass container again and again with water as well as the pink salt rocks, continuing the process.

This brime is also recommended for gargling. It balances the pH in your mouth and works against gum bleeding, canker sores and bad breath. (Combine with one capful of natural mouthwash, one capful of hydrogen peroxide, and 5-6 squirts of SonicSilver™. Brush your teeth with a natural toothpaste for an even more dramatic result. Done consistently, your teeth will become whiter and tartar will dissolve.

How Andes Pink Salt Compares

How does the Andes pink salt compare to the common poison we call table salt? Andes pink salt is health-supporting. It is not bitter but has a robust flavor for cooking (I put a pinch of it in everything I eat). Andes pink salt is not contaminated by pollution or heavy metals. This salt has one of the highest amounts of alkalizing-minerals compared to than any other salt or sea salt.

It provides:

1. Calcium
2. Potassium
3. Magnesium

You can use Andes pink salt for:

1. A table salt for cooking

2. Salt bathing to recover from fatigue
3. Drinking a mild-salt solution (Brim) to balance the body
4. Gargling, especially when fighting a cold
5. Brushing teeth to help fight gum disease
6. Rinsing nasal passages (as with a Neti pot wash)

22 THINGS SEAWATER OR SEA SALT IS GOOD FOR

1. Salt is most effective in stabilizing irregular heartbeats and, contrary to the misconception that it causes high blood pressure, it is actually essential for the regulation of blood pressure – in conjunction with water. Naturally the proportions are critical.
2. Salt is vital to the extraction of excess acidity from the cells in the body, particularly the brain cells.
3. Salt is vital for balancing the sugar levels in the blood; a needed element in treating diabetes.
4. Salt is vital for the generation of hydroelectric energy in cells in the body. It is used for local power generation at the sites of energy needed by the cells.
5. Salt is vital to communication between nerve cells.
6. Salt is vital for absorption of food particles through the intestinal tract.
7. Salt is vital for the clearance of the lungs of mucus plugs and sticky phlegm, particularly in asthma and cystic fibrosis.
8. Salt is vital for clearing up catarrh (inflammation of the mucus

membranes) and congestion of the sinuses.

9. Salt is a strong natural antihistamine.
10. Salt is essential for the prevention of muscle cramps.
11. Salt is vital for preventing excess saliva production (a condition where it would flow out of the mouth during sleep). If you need to constantly mop up excess saliva, this indicates a salt shortage.
12. Salt is absolutely vital to making the structure of bones firm. Osteoporosis, in a major way, is a result of salt and water shortages in the body.
13. Salt is vital for sleep regulation. It is a natural hypnotic.
14. Salt on the tongue will stop persistent dry coughs.
15. Salt is vital for the prevention of gout and gouty arthritis.
16. Salt is vital for maintaining sexuality and libido.
17. Salt is vital for preventing varicose veins and spider veins on the legs and thighs.
18. Salt is vital to the information-processing brain cells do, from the moment of conception to death.
19. Salt is vital for reducing a double chin. When the body is short of salt, it means the body really is short of water. The salivary glands sense the salt shortage and are obliged to produce more saliva to lubricate the act of chewing and swallowing and also to supply the stomach with water that it needs for breaking down foods. Circulation to the salivary glands increases and the blood vessels become "leaky" in order to supply the glands with water to manufacture saliva. The "leakiness" spills beyond the area of the glands themselves, causing increased bulk under the skin of the chin, the cheeks and into the neck.
20. Sea salt contains about 80 mineral elements that the body needs. Some of these elements are needed in trace amounts. Unrefined sea salt is a better choice of salt than other types of salt on the market. Ordinary table salt that is bought in the supermarkets has been stripped of its companion elements and contains additive elements such as aluminum silicate to keep it powdery and easy to pour. Aluminum is a very toxic element to our nervous system. It is implicated as one of the primary causes of Alzheimer's disease.
21. Twenty-seven percent of the body's salt is in the bones. Osteoporosis results when the body needs more salt and takes it from the body. Bones are 22% water. Is it not obvious what happens to the bones when we're deficient in salt or water or both?

Gee Wiz:
Why are we told it should be a low-salt or no-salt diet? As you have witnessed, pure salt is essential to life.

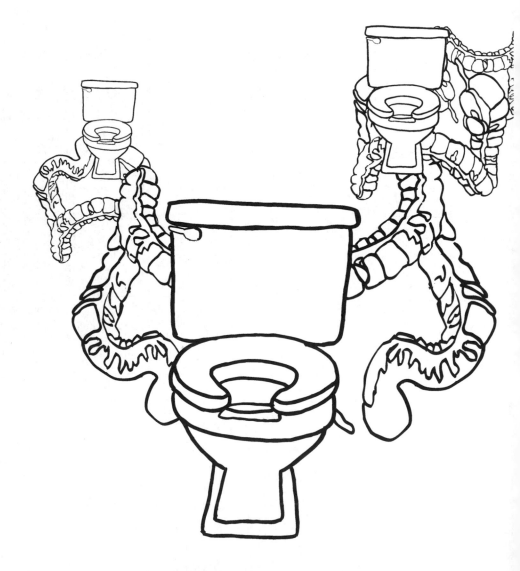

CHAPTER 10

The Trend of the Evil, Uncharted Wind (Gas)

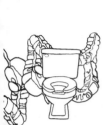

Surely, we know that the "art of the fart" will release inhibitions in a previously on-going conversation. So simply say, "Excuse me, but I must mix this gas with some fresh air." Then step outside. No big deal, but please step outside.

WHAT IS GAS (FLATULENCE)?

Although embarrassing and most times stinky, passing gas is a completely natural human process. It's caused by eating and digesting, and the chemical reactions of carbohydrates, proteins, fats and other hard-to-digest foods. Certain gasses can blister paint on walls and cause house plants to wilt. What is your gas of choice?

UNDIGESTED CARBOHYDRATES

When you eat, the food reaches the stomach, and it is digested or broken down into a liquid through chemical actions caused by acids and enzymes. Most carbohydrates are certainly broken down in this way. However, some complex carbohydrates (which are found in a vast array of grains, vegetables and some fruits) escape this and end up in the intestinal track in various states of being less than fully processed. That's when the fun begins.

When the partially digested carbs reach the colon, there are a multitude of bacteria waiting to get down and feast on these leftovers. One of the by-products of foods lingering in the colon is *GAS*. The colon doesn't have teeth; it cannot chew undigested foods. Nor does it have the proper enzymes to break down the foods. These foods sit in that nice hot pool of bacteria and they ferment (picture yeast, mold, germs, parasites and heat). It's hot in there! Fermenting is a *GAS!* So Chew, Chew, Chew, and then Chew some more.

GAS IS ALSO A BY-PRODUCT OF OUR OTHER HABITS, ETC.

1. **CHEWING GUM.** You're swallowing air – GAS.
2. **CARBONATED DRINKS** (sodas). You're swallowing air – GAS.
3. **POOR FOOD-COMBINING.** You eat protein and follow that with sweet cake – GAS.
4. **TALKING & EATING AT THE SAME TIME.** You're gulping air – GAS.
5. **OVERLOAD OF PARASITES.** There's decomposing debris in there – GAS.
6. **YOU'RE OVER-EATING PROTEIN.** There's too much in the pipeline, and it's undergoing putrefaction – GAS.
7. **UNCHEWED FRUITS, VEGGIES, WHATEVER!** You're eating too fast – GAS.
8. **NEGLECTING TO TAKE A PROBIOTIC.** You can win the battle between the Good and Bad Bacteria by giving the good guys some support. (See the next chapter.)

Actually, sometimes I think that I won't be surprised if certain folks would just spontaneously combust!

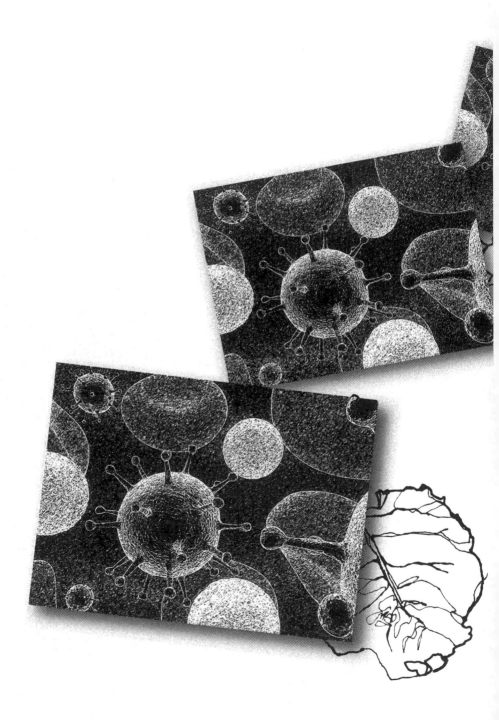

CHAPTER 11

Bacteria: The Good, the Bad, the Ugly

It is essential to replace the good bacteria following a colonic and just as important following antibiotics. Allow me to explain …

Probiotics, aka "The Good," are also known as "friendly bacteria." They are a part of our intestinal flora. In fact, according to leading researcher Khem Shahani, PhD, there are **billions** of microorganisms living in our gastrointestinal tract. The majority of these organisms are bacteria, and there are also fungi (yeast) and protozoa. You may know good bacteria as **acidophilus,** an active ingredient in many yogurts.

Probiotic literally means "Anything that supports life" while antibiotic means "Destructive of life." You know that antibiotics are drugs administered for the purpose of killing off infectious bacteria that cause illness and symptoms of illness. However, what you may not realize is that antibiotics kill off the bacteria whether it is good or bad.

So you have a bacterial illnesses, and you take an antibiotic which immediately kills all the bacteria (remember, both the Good and the Bad). This puts the bad bacteria in check for the moment and most times symptoms disappear. However, probiotics should then be introduced to re-colonize the good bacteria (which was killed off). That way, you will return your body to homeostasis (balance). As you take the probiotics on a daily basis, the friendly bacteria will continue to hold any bad bacteria that grow in check and under-thumb.

RECAP: *Following antibiotics, take pro-biotics.* That is not at the same time, but afterwards. In the next chapter, you'll find information on my **Inner Body Bath Probiotic.** Its active ingredient is *Lactobacillus sporogenes,* a universally-occurring beneficial bacteria.

BAD BACTERIA WILL WEAKEN THE IMMUNE SYSTEM!

Key to a healthy body is balance (homeostasis). Only 15-20% putrefactive bacteria (such as *E. coli, B. putreficus, B. welchii,* etc.) should exist in your pre-cious body. These detrimental bacteria produce toxins and gas. Let's face it … they are nasty critters.

FRIENDLY BACTERIA SUPPORT & STRENGTHEN YOUR IMMUNITY!

The colon contains about 500 variet-ies of bacteria. The friendly bacteria (including *L. acidophilus, L. bifidus, L. bulgaricus, L. salivarius, L. sporogenes,* etc.) should maintain 80-85% occupancy for balance.

THAT'S THE GOOD & BAD; HERE'S THE *UGLY*

With the Standard American Diet (SAD) and use of antibiotics, the balance of your precious body can switch from 80-85% friendly bacteria to a whop-ping 80-90% un-friendly bacteria. Now you're an accident waiting to happen. And for some, this accident will spring up like a surprise party from the first ring in hell … Suddenly you'll find yourself in a disease crisis.

CAUSE OF A TOXIC POLLUTED DISTORTED COLON

Harmful bacteria, parasites and worms hang out in a polluted colon, where they thrive on the filth, the rotting, stag-nant putrefying matter, the stinky and fermenting carbohydrates.

The body can be like a walking gar-bage can, carrying that rotting matter in the colon for extended periods. In this state, as an old Arabic saying tells us, "The gut is the father of all afflictions." However, your bowel can normally carry out its proper function of effi-ciently eliminating waste and absorbing nutrients. Its original natural design is remarkable and extremely efficient. But important to good health and healing, you must allow friendly bacteria to remain well colonized.

The BAD bacteria support the backing up and holding on of unwanted matter. Keep in mind that unfriendly bacteria are living critters and require food to live. When you consume animal protein, unnecessary sugars, processed foods and the like, you are feeding the little nasties.

There is absolutely no doubt that fol-lowing a good bowel movement, you feel so great! Your senses are keener, the feeling of being bloated has sub-sided. The sky is clear (and it's raining outside!) and you're singing opera. It's a beautiful thing. Well, in addition to warding off an overgrowth of the bad bacteria, probiotics can also help you become "regular." It's amazing what a difference probiotics can make!

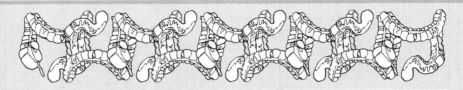

Scary Colon Cancer Statistics*

In 2009, 10% of all cancer-related deaths were due to colon and rectum cancer.

- 1 in 18 men will develop colon or rectum cancer.

- 1 in 20 women will develop colon or rectum cancer.

"Colon cancer does not care about age, sex, education or income level. Cancer can strike anyone at anytime," says a CDC press release.

* These stats are from the Centers for Disease Control & Prevention (CDC).

Not enough attention is paid to this area of the body until a crisis ensues. Then it may be too late!

If your doctor ignores your humongous, ginormous belly, he or she knows you are future money. The bigger your belly, the more waste you are storing.

This is toxic waste. *It will kill you.* If not directly, than indirectly … but it will kill you.

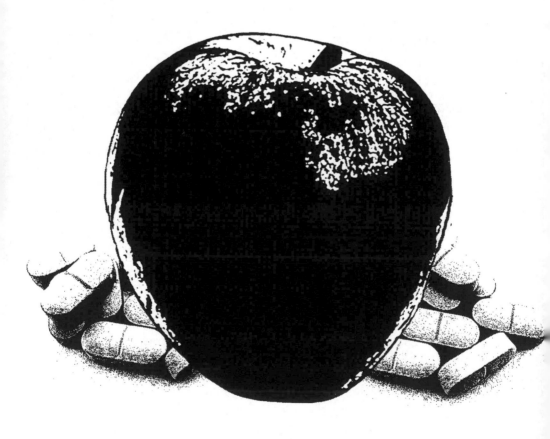

CHAPTER 12

Health Helpers: Supplements, Products & More

Years ago, we used to be able to get away with not taking supplements. However, we can't do that today with our current onslaught of toxins, stressful lifestyles, and degraded soils for agriculture. This chapter will highlight the supplements and products I most often recommend to my clients at the Life Well Institute.

As you saw in the "Walking My Talk" chapter (Chapter 6), I have devised my personal health regimen over the years. With my work as a colon hydrotherapist, I am exposed to cutting-edge supplements and the best approaches for care that the alternative world of health has to offer. I am pleased to be able to share this info with you through my book *The Body Doesn't Know How to Die.*

Note: Most of the supplements and products mentioned in this chapter can be ordered through my website, http://www.indiashealthyliving.com/.

intraMAX, a Liquid Multi-mineral with Vitamins

This supplement is a 100%-organic liquid blend of 415+ nutrients. Drucker Labs' **intraMAX** provides 71+ full-spectrum trace minerals, 64 vitamins, 124 antioxidants, 40 amino acids, seven essential fatty acids, 14 digestive enzymes, 13 probiotics, 43 super green foods/phytonutrients, and more. I like **intraMAX** because it is scientifically advanced and clinically proven to be health-promoting. It is made with a proprietary organic "carbon-bond" intracell technology which enables the nutrients to be absorbed more readily by your cells.

This is the basic daily supplement that I recommend. It is a 100% natural, vegetarian supplement, with no additives. Note that physicians recommend *intraMAX* to their pregnant clients because it is an excellent product and easier to swallow than prenatal vitamins. For me, liquid supplements are my first choice because they are quickly absorbed into your system.

You must call Drucker Labs (1-888-881-2344) for your initial order. This product is only sold through healthcare practitioners. So introduce your healthcare provider to *intraMAX,* the best multi-mineral on the market. Or you can use my ID Number H017300 to order it directly.

Common dosage of *intraMAX* is one ounce. For best results, take on an empty stomach. Do not take within 2 hours of pharmaceuticals, nutraceuticals and/or OTC medications. If possible, hold the product under your tongue for 60 seconds before swallowing. If you have sensitive teeth or gums, swallow immediately. After swallowing, sip 8 to 10 ounces of alkaline water or spring water with lemon. Not recommended after 6 p.m.

INNER BODY BATH PROBIOTIC

Most probiotics must be refrigerated or they will lose their potency. However no refrigeration is needed for my *Inner Body Bath Probiotic.* Take it on a regular basis or particularly right after antibiotic treatment to maintain a healthy amount of friendly bacteria in your system. I also recommend that you take probiotics after a colon hydrotherapy session.

The probiotic in this supplement is L. sporogenes, which has the ability to be successfully implanted in the intestines. The supplement also contains the prebiotic FOS (FructoOligoSaccharides), which serves as a food source for the beneficial bacteria in the colon. Other ingredients are ginger (which is soothing to the digestive tract) and flax seed (an insoluble fiber). Adults and children over 16 take 1-2 capsules daily or an amount recommended by their healthcare practitioner.

INNER BODY BATH REAL EASEZYME

Digestive enzymes help the body break down food more effectively so that it can be well digested. My *Inner Body Bath Real EaseZyme* contains four types of enzymes: (1) Amylase, for carbohydrates, starches and sugars; (2) Lipase, for the fats in oils, dairy, nuts and meats; (3) Cellulase, for plant fiber including cellulose, and (4) Protease, for the protein in meats, eggs, cheese and nuts. In addition to the enzymes, it also provides an herbal formula that assists the body

Important Note

It is important to speak to your healthcare provider before taking any supplement. For the best results, inquire first before trying the supplements.

FROM ARTICLES.MERCOLA.COM

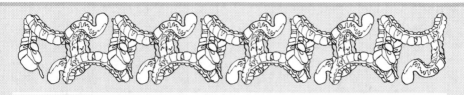

Herbal Ingredients in *Dr. Schulze Formula #1*

Curaçao and Cape Aloe Leaf, Senna Leaf and Pod, Cascara Sagrada Aged Bark, Oregon Grape Root, Hawaiian Yellow Ginger Root, Garlic Bulb, and Habanero Peppers.

Herbal Ingredients in *Dr. Schulze Formula #2*

Flax Seed, Psyllium Seed, Apple Pectin, Activated Willow Charcoal, Marshmallow Root, Pharmaceutical Grade Bentonite Clay, Slippery Elm Bark, Peppermint Leaf and Cayenne Pepper Blend.

in moving food through your system. Two capsules are taken between meals and/or just before bed with adequate liquid. In addition to supporting digestion, enzymes can also be helpful for reducing inflammation – including inflamed joints.

DR. SCHULZE COLON CLEANSING FORMULAS

For products specifically for colon cleansing, I turn to formulas from Dr. Richard Schulze. Dr. Schulze's own health challenge at age 14 (a heart defect) led him to explore the best of what the world of alternative therapies had to offer. After regaining his health, Dr. Schulze became a master herbalist and obtained other degrees – eventually treating tens of thousands of patients over three decades.

The colon cleansing supplements that I recommend are *Dr. Schulze's Intestinal Formula #1* and *Intestinal Formula #2*. *Formula #1* promotes healthy bowel movements and stimulates peristalsis (contractions of the colon walls that move matter onward). *Formula #2* helps draw out stored fecal matter, as well as toxins, heavy metals, and unhealthy bacteria.

Bowel Flush Shot

Dr. Richard Schulze says that he has learned a few things over the three decades at his clinic. One is that as humans we are not perfect. Thus *Dr. Schulze's Bowel Flush Shot* was devised for those times when you've indulged in the wrong foods, and are now feeling miserable and clogged up. At my clinic, I consider this to be a supplement to use in "emergencies." For instance, let's say that you've been traveling, eating different foods, and you've become constipated. You haven't pooped in three days, and you'd like to get things moving again. I refer to the *Bowel Flush Shot* as the "Master Blaster." The Schulze company says that it will empty your bowels and digestive system by the following morning, in some cases in 2 hours. It's smart to take the package of three shots along on a trip. A typical dosage is taking an individual solo shot, the second shot 2 hours later, and the third shot 2 hours after that.

In addition to your own healthcare provider, you can also get support from the staff at Dr. Schulze (1-800-HERB-DOC) when using their products.

SONIC SILVER

This is a natural alternative to antibiotics which contains 99.9999% pure natural ionic silver mineral particles. It is a

---

Herbal Ingredients in the *Bowel Flush Shot*

Dr. Schulze's Proprietary Cathartic Formula: Senna Leaf and Pod, Cascara Sagrada Aged Bark; Dr. Schulze's Proprietary Carminative Formula: Hawaiian Yellow Ginger Root, Peppermint Leaf and Oil, and Anise Seed; Dr. Schulze's Proprietary WormEx Formula: Agrimony Herb, Black Walnut Hulls, Cinchona Bark, Clove Bud, Goldenseal Root, and Thyme Leaf.

---

multi-purpose germ fighter that you can spray on your body or on any surface that you touch and want to be germ-free. Colloidal silver used to be the antibiotic of choice in doctor's offices, but later it went out of fashion. According to the manufacturer of *Sonic Silver,* the product has been used successfully with infections, athlete's foot, yeast infections and rashes. *Sonic Silver* also comes in a nasal spray that includes eucalyptus extract. The nasal spray was formulated to bring relief from clogged and stuffy nasal passages due to allergies or infection.

I use *Sonic Silver* daily to keep my immune system strong. In my practice, I encounter people with colds or flu often, and I am rarely sick. *Sonic Silver* can be sprayed under the tongue or on the tonsils. For my patients, I recommend it only be taken when fighting off infections or in place of antibiotics.

KARISALT ANDES PINK (SEA) SALT

The best salt by far is *Karisalt's Andes Pink (Sea) Salt.* It was formed over three hundred million years ago. A pure deep ocean evaporated, and the salt was buried under the Andes Mountains, which protected this reserve from pollutants. The incredible weight of the mountains over long periods of time transformed the salt into a very special form of crystallized rock salt. Andes pink salt has no sediment, and it is not refined. It is mined, crushed and delivered in a natural state.

For information on a daily health routine using *Andes Pink Salt,* see the "Blood, Sweat and Tears" chapter (Chapter 9).

MY 90-DAY CANDIDA CONTROL PROGRAM

Candida Albicans is a naturally-occurring yeast that is found in moist areas of the human body. When the natural balance of the body is upset (perhaps by antibiotics, stress or poor diet [high-sugar or high-carbohydrate eating]), the changing internal environment may allow this yeast to overgrow. Not only may the yeast increase in areas where it is normally found (the vagina/genitals, gastrointestinal tract, mouth and throat). The opportunistic yeast may leak through the intestinal walls into the bloodstream, and then travel to other parts of the body. Now we have a problem. It's called Candida or a yeast infection.

Symptoms of a yeast overgrowth include:

- Gas and bloating
- Fatigue
- Itching
- Brain fog
- Headaches
- Skin conditions

Over time, excess Candida may lead to Irritable Bowel Syndrome, Depression, Chronic Fatigue, Multiple Chemical Sensitivity Syndrome, Fibromyalgia, Food Allergies, Muscle and Joint Pain, etc.

Because of all the potential problems, it is wise to nip a Candida overgrowth in the bud as soon as possible. One very effective way is with my 90-Day Candida Control Program.

Everyone is unique. The 90-Day Program to control Candida will affect each individual differently, with varying results. Most people feel healthier at the end of the 90 days.

There are two supplements used in this program:

1. *Inner Body Bath Probiotic*
2. *Candida-G* (Candida Natural Anti-Fungal & Probiotic + Aloe)

My *Inner Body Bath Probiotic*, which was described earlier in this chapter, is used orally to fight to control the Candida. The active ingredient, L. Sporogenes, helps restore a healthy balance of microflora in your body. Thus the beneficial bacteria help control the Candida (yeast).

The *Candida-G* also contains L. sporogenes, along with Aloe Vera. It can be used both internally or topically. The combination of the L. Sporogenes with the Aloe Vera creates a synergy of power to identify and control the Candida.

During the 90-Day Protocol, drink a lot of water. As your body detoxifies, you may experience aches and pains, stiffness of the joints, and skin rashes. This is called a "yeast die-off." If you experience such effects, you have a choice of reducing your daily dose for a couple days, or pushing through it and moving on with the higher dosage.

Suggested daily dosage:

First day: Take one capsule of the *Candida-G* at bedtime.

Second day: Take one capsule of the *Candida-G* in the morning and take one capsule of the *Inner Body Bath Probiotic* before going to bed.

Third day: Take one capsule of the *Candida-G* and one capsule of the *Inner Body Bath Probiotic* in the morning. Before bed, take one more capsule of the *Inner Body Bath Probiotic.*

Fourth day: Take one capsule of the *Candida-G* and three capsules of the *Inner Body Bath Probiotic.*

Fifth day: Take one capsule of the *Candida-G* and four capsules of the *Inner Body Bath Probiotic.*

Sixth & Seventh day: Take three capsules of the *Inner Body Bath Probiotic* only.

Eighth day: Start the process again. Continue this program for two weeks, and then reduce to the maintenance dosage and continue for 90 days. The **maintenance dosage** is two *Inner Body Bath Probiotics* daily and two *Candida-Gs* every other day for the remainder of the 90 days after the initial two week program.

With this regimen you can include *Sonic Silver,* the natural alternative to antibiotics described above. You can spray it on your hair and on other areas where the yeast are causing a problem.

Bowel movements which increase in volume will be your first indicator that this regimen is working. After seven days, you can continue with this protocol, or either increase or decrease the dosage of the products. You must learn to read your body. In times of increased stress, increase the dosage.

Topical: Add one capsule of *Candida-G* into 4-6 ounces of water. For best results, use a spray bottle. Apply and rub into the skin firmly. If using on the hair, apply after a shower and let it soak in. Observe the results wherever it is applied. The liquid for spraying will last three to four days. When treating the hair, pour it on your head the last day, rub it in, and then shower.

Women: Spray the *Candida-G* mixture on your face in the morning before you apply your make-up. Yeast can actually get into and live in your make-up. Also, spray your face with the mixture after you remove your make-up.

THE WONDERS OF AMINO ACIDS

Amino acids are commonly described as "the building blocks of protein." When we eat a protein, the digestive system breaks the food down into its constituent amino acids. There are a total of 20 different kinds of amino acids derived from protein.

Supplementation with amino acids can have many positive effects on the body and psyche. Author Julia Ross has written extensively on this topic in her books, *The Diet Cure* and *The Mood Cure.* I highly recommend both titles.

Over the years, I've worked with Ross's ideas and done further research to develop different combinations of supplements that include amino acids. I offer two basic Amino Acid Protocols in this chapter.

Amino Acid Combo One

L-Glutamine

5-HTP

DL Phenylalanine

Plus (if emphasis is more energy):

Chromium

B complex

Let's look at each of these supplements separately.

L-Glutamine: This amino acid is important for repair of the intestinal walls, such as in cases of leaky gut. Providing glycogen, it helps restore energy. It also assists in maintaining cell health, and thus speeds up healing.

5-HTP: This is a naturally occurring amino acid, as well as a chemical byproduct of the amino acid L-tryptophan. People take it for a variety of conditions, including depression and anxiety, as well as sleep disorders.

DL Phenylalaline: This is a combination of L-Phenylalanine (a naturally occurring amino acid) and D-Phenylalanine (a version of L-Phenylalanine synthesized in labs). Most often, it is used to address nerve health and improve mood.

Chromium: This is a mineral which we need in trace amounts. Chromium enhances the processing of insulin, and it supports metabolism. A lack of chromium can impair our ability to use glucose for energy needs. Currently there is research interest in chromium's ability to correct glucose intolerance and insulin resistance, conditions that can lead to diabetes.

B complex: A B complex supplement includes B1 (thiamine), B2 (riboflavin), B3 (niacin), B5 (pantothenic acid), B6 (pyridoxine), biotin, folic acid and B12 (the cobalamins). Each substance has its own unique role in the body. Together they are taken to strengthen the blood, address skin conditions, support the assimilation of food, and the conversion of carbohydrates for energy.

At my clinic, I use Combo One to improve the everyday experience of my clients. This combination helps to regulate the body's temperature (if you happen to be someone who feels too hot one moment, and too cold the next). It improves the wake/sleep cycle as well. It also helps reduce sugar cravings.

Amino Acid Combo Two

This two supplement combo is good alone to reduce sugar cravings:

L-Glutamine

Alpha Lorporic Acid

L-Glutamine: See background above.

Alpha Lorporic Acid: This is a super antioxidant, a substance that can neutralize free radicals. It is also a fatty acid found in every cell. It helps the body produce energy from blood sugar (so it is a great help in balancing blood sugar levels).

Excess sugar has profound negative effects on your body. It depresses the immune system. It contributes to cancers of the breast, colon and reproductive organs. It speeds aging. It messes with your blood sugar, and can lead to cycles of extreme highs and lows. According in Julia Ross, sugar is also a key player in the development of heart disease.

For further background on sugar cravings and the dangers of sugar, read the classic health book *Sugar Blues* by William F. Duffy.

At the clinic, I adapt the amino acid regimens for the individual. So you can try one of these combinations, do more of your own research for what you might need, or come in to see me. There is additional information on using amino acids in the "sugar cravings" section of the diet chapter (Chapter 8).

Caution: Per Julia Ross's *Mood Cure* site, it is especially important to consult a qualified healthcare professional before taking any amino acids if you have a serious physical illness, such as cancer. If you have an overactive thyroid, PKU (phenylketonuria), or melanoma, she says not to take DL-Phenylalanine. For additional precautions, visit http:/www.moodcure.com/aminoacidprecautions.html.

REAL FOOD, REAL LIFE™ FERMENTED PRODUCTS

Over the years, many health authorities have noticed that cultures that eat a regular diet of fermented foods seem to live longer lives and to experience extended good health. An intake of a simple diet that includes predigested protein has helped them to hold on to their health and vitality. Real Food, Real Life products contain a fermented powder that is a predigested form of protein, carbohydrate and fatty acids. This powder helps the body digest food more efficiently. It also provides all the necessary amino acids, which are the building blocks of protein and important for repair and maintenance of the human body. The company uses an ancient fermentation process that they have refined and improved upon. They call it the FermFlora process. This process also creates a naturally occurring predigested probiotic.

Real Food, Real Life's botanical probiotic supplements include:

Pro-Daily-Otic (powder)

Pro-Amino-Otic (powder)

Great Grains Pro-Belly-Otic (liquid)

Grapefruit Pro-Belly-Otic (liquid)

Lime-Mint Pro-Belly-Otic (liquid)

Green Rhino Energy Probiotic (liquid – includes fermented guarana for an energy boost)

For more information, go to my site and click on the Real Food, Real Life link.

ISAGENIX INTERNATIONAL

Another excellent company for supplements is Isagenix of Chandler, Arizona. One Isagenix product that I recommend is their meal replacement shake, *IsaLean*. An *IsaLean* shake contains 23 grams of high-quality whey and casein protein, along with healthy fats and energy-boosting carbohydrates. This drink is low in saturated fat, sodium and cholesterol, and it contains only 240 calories and 6 grams of fat. Available in chocolate and vanilla, it comes in liquid form so no mixing is necessary. *IsaLean* is clinically proven to support weight loss and weight management. You can use the shake to replace one to two meals when on a weight loss program.

Another handy Isagenix product is their *Want More Energy?* drink powder. This product supplies a natural energy boost from B vitamins and minerals. The powder comes in a canister of 45 servings and a box of 36 sticks (individually packaged servings that can be added to 16 ounces of water). *Want More Energy?* is available in the following flavors: orange, grape or citrus, or in a mixed box of sticks.

YOUR GRANDMOTHER'S REMEDY, CASTOR OIL

Castor oil has been turned to throughout the ages as a natural therapy. The matriarchs in my childhood neighborhood used it as a common remedy. This is a vegetable oil that comes from the castor bean, which technically is the castor seed.

Using Castor Oil Packs

Today, applying castor oil externally in the form of "packs" is a very popular approach with natural health practitioners. The Edgar Cayce Readings tell us that castor oil packs are to be used to improve assimilations, eliminations and circulation (especially of the lymphatic system). William A. McGarey, MD, author of *The Oil that Heals,* used Cayce's methods for 30 years, and he found castor oil relieved pain, helped the body to heal, and stimulated immunity. It will also rouse the bowel.

A castor oil pack is often made of several layers of wool flannel material, enough to absorb and hold the castor oil during application. Using either wool flannel or cotton flannel is a personal choice. Some individuals are sensitive to wool.

A common area to apply the castor oil pack is on the right side of the abdomen, between the upper part of the rib cage and the upper edge of the hipbone.

Another common area is across the abdomen from the right to the left side of the body, covering from the sternum (also called the "breast bone") to the pubic or groin area.

Application is usually for one to two hours. A hot water bottle or buckwheat pillow is placed on top of the castor oil pack to keep it warm during application. I don't recommend a heating pad because it gives off too much electromagnetic radiation (EMF). You can consult your health practitioner to determine the frequency of application for a particular condition.

You can protect your hot water bottle by using plastic wrap. Fold the flannel wool (or cotton wool) into two to three layers. Add castor oil to the fabric a little at a time, saturating all three layers, but not so much that it drips from the flannel. Place the flannel on the top of the hot water bottle for about 1-3 minutes or until the oil is warm. Place a large old towel across the area where you're going to lie down. When you are ready to begin, flip the castor oil pack and hot water bottle onto your abdomen area so the flannel is against your skin. Fold the ends of the towel (that's underneath you) over the hot water bottle and relax. If desired, you can fasten the towel snugly with large safety pins. Again, a session is usually for an hour or two.

After the session, a solution of 2 teaspoons of baking soda mixed into one quart of water can be used to clean your skin.

After three days of using the castor oil pack, take about 1 teaspoon of olive oil (NOT castor oil) by mouth in the evening before retiring.

You can use the same castor oil pack for additional applications. It is important to discard the pack after a certain number of uses or before it becomes rancid. It may be helpful to store the pack in a plastic storage container and refrigerate between uses. The wool and cotton flannel packs can be used for approximately 25-30 applications before they are to be discarded.

Cold-pressed castor oil is available in 8-ounce, pint, or gallon-size containers. Frequent users usually purchase it by the gallon. Small amounts of castor oil should be added to the pack before each use to refresh it.

Taking Castor Oil by Mouth

Taken internally, castor oil acts like a laxative. Make no mistake about it. Castor oil is very effective for emptying the bowel. About a tablespoon or two will stimulate the emptying of the entire bowel, within about five hours. This is a serious old remedy from hundreds of years ago. It worked then, and it will work now. Because some cramping and discomfort can occur, I prefer

Important Note

Always seek medical advice prior to use of castor oil. Do NOT use castor oil packs during pregnancy or during menstrual flow.

that my clients use the *Dr. Schulze Bowel Flush Shot.*

Castor Oil Massage

Castor oil can be massaged on the abdomen to lubricate the intestines when someone is constipated. It is soothing, as well as stimulating to the bowel. This is a gentler approach than taking the castor oil by mouth. I suggest this to mothers who come in with children who have been constipated. Check with your pediatrician to get his/her input before trying this approach.

As Part of My Total Body Detox

With the "India's Total Body Detox" treatment at the clinic, I incorporate castor oil packs into a two-hour session that also includes jumping on a rebounder (small trampoline), soaking in a whirlpool hydro tub, lymphatic drainage massage, foot detox, and a colonic. This is a great cleanse, and it helps people who have been experiencing constipation. Usually they will release the matter after the first time I fill them up with water during the colonic. Then when I fill them up a second time, the water is able to hydrate their colon and their system.

Note: Castor oil is available through neighborhood drugstores.

HELPFUL PRODUCTS

African Red Tea®

Rooibos African Red Tea has 50 times more antioxidants than green tea. It contains the minerals iron, potassium, calcium, copper, zinc, magnesium, manganese and sodium. This tea is great tasting and naturally sweet. The flavor is full-bodied and extremely smooth. *African Red Tea* is 100% organic and caffeine-free. It comes in a box of 20 tea bags. This is a great tea that's good for the body and soul. As an adaptogen, it is able to refresh you throughout your day and then relax you when you're ready for sleep.

SereniGy Coffee

I am not an advocate of coffee drinking. However, if you must drink coffee, this is the one I would recommend. SereniGy Gourmet Coffee, a great tasting cup of Joe with a smooth flavor, is a blend that includes 100% certified organic Ganoderma. A highly nutritious herb, Ganoderma has been used for 4000 years in Traditional Chinese Medicine. Known as the "King of Herbs," it is turned to for its ability to promote longevity, help restore balance to the body, enable the body to endure various types of stress, and support the immune system. Ganoderma is also a fatigue fighter, and it has antioxidant properties.

The company developed this product in a way that would deliver the fullest spectrum of nutrients possible from the Ganoderma. This herb is known as "Ling zhi" in China and "Reishi" in Japan (yes, like the medicinal mushrooms). In China, it is widely used in many different types of products.

To order the coffee and for more info, go to www.serenigy.com/mmorales. Enter the ID# 100200 to place an order.

Footstool for the Toilet

Have you ever heard that human beings weren't built to sit on a throne to do our business in the bathroom, but rather it would be more natural for us to squat? When we're seated, our anal canal is not straight, but rather it's a bit choked. All that you might need to have a smoother elimination is a small footstool under your feet to mimic the squatting position when you're on the toilet.

This may sound odd to you, but a footstool will really make it easier for you to make a deposit in the bathroom. You most likely won't have to strain; it will just flow.

The *HealthStep* is the brand of bathroom footstool that I recommend. It is available through my website.

Conclusion

As mentioned earlier, most of the supplements and products in this chapter are conveniently available through my website, www.indiashealthyliving.com. Stop by and go to the "Shop" section of the site to see all that is available and to check out pricing.

When it comes to supplements, we're not talking about being on life support 24/7. But know that there is natural support available for your body as you work on maintaining or restoring your good health. Check them out, for the health of it!

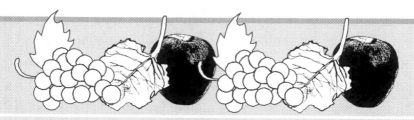

RECIPES

These awesome, healthy and great-tasting recipes were created by Niambi Sims, Owner of Integrated Wellness Concepts (www.integratedwellnessconcepts.com).

Sautéed Green Beans and Mushrooms

10 Crimini (common) or Oyster mushrooms
2 Handfuls of green beans
1 Bunch of scallions sliced
1/4 Cup of olive oil

1. Heat 2 quarts water to boil. Add beans, cook for five minutes and set aside.

2. Heat olive oil in a sauté pan, then add the mushrooms and scallions. Stir for two minutes. Add beans, season to your preference and serve as a side dish.

Stir-Fry Greens

3 Bunches of greens* cut in strips
1 Red or green bell pepper cut in strips
1/2 Tablespoon of chopped garlic
1/4 Cup of teriyaki sauce or Bragg's Liquid Aminos
1 Tablespoon of agave nectar
2 Tablespoons olive oil

1. Heat a wok or sauté pan, then add oil. Throw in the garlic and the greens; stir for three minutes.

2. Lower heat, and add red or green pepper, and agave nectar. Also add the teriyaki sauce or Bragg's Liquid Aminos. Cook five more minutes, then serve.

*Turnip Greens, Collards, Kale, Chard or Mustard Greens.

GREEN SMOOTHIE

1 Handful of kale
1/2 Ripe banana
1 c Apple juice
1/2 Apple
1 teaspoon of powdered flax seed

Add all ingredients into a blender and blend until smooth. Enjoy!

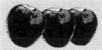

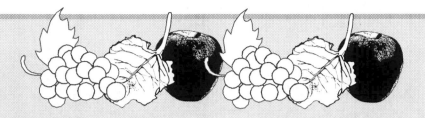

Spaghetti Squash Marinara

1   Spaghetti squash
2   Roma tomatoes
1   Onion
1   Teaspoon chopped garlic
1-2 Cups marinara sauce
2   Tablespoons olive oil
1/2 Teaspoon of salt
1   Handful of fresh basil (optional)
*   Parmesan cheese (optional)

1. Slice the squash in half.

2. Place both halves face down on lightly greased baking pan.

3. Bake for 30 minutes.

4. Meanwhile in a sauce pan, heat the oil. Add garlic, onion, basil, tomatoes and salt. Sauté for 3 minutes

5. Heat marinara sauce.

5. Remove squash and let cool.

6. With a large spoon, scoop out strands of squash into a large mixing bowl.

7. Add sautéed tomato mixture into bowl; mix thoroughly.

8. Serve squash onto serving plates, and add marinara sauce on top. Garnish with Parmesan and fresh basil leaves.

Stone Fruit Salad

2   Ripe peaches
1   Ripe nectarine
2   Plums
1/4 Cup agave nectar or honey
1   Pinch of allspice
1   Pinch of anise
1/4 Cup of water

1. Pit fruit and cut into bite-sized chunks.
2. Mix honey, water, allspice and anise into bowl.
3. Add fruit to mixture. Toss and serve.

Cranberry Spinach Salad

2   Bunches of spinach (or one bag)
1/4 Cup dried cranberries
1/3 Cup slivered almonds
1/4 Cup apple cider vinegar
1/4 Cup olive oil
1   Pinch of salt

1. In a large bowl, mix spinach, cranberries and almonds.
2. In a separate bowl, mix vinegar, salt and oil.
3. Mix dressing into salad (to taste).

Acknowledgments

The intention and inspiration to write this book was encouraged by my many faithful clients over many years who insisted that I put my teachings in writing. It has been, in fact, a learning experience for me. Thank you all so very much.

I would especially like to thank the Cerritos Center for the Performing Arts (CCPA). "Why CCPA," you ask? As a healer, it is extremely difficult to maintain a positive attitude when in the presence of those who either do not feel well or their energy is so low 24/7. I've always said, "Stress alone can kill you," and CCPA has been my stress relief. I have enjoyed the entertainment and cultural enrichment found there, and I would have burned out long ago and this book would not have been possible without my part-time work at the Center. My co-workers at CCPA are my extended family, and CCPA's seasonal supporters and donors including some of the administrative staff at the Life Well Institute, and many of my friends and associates as well. But most of all I send appreciation to the CCPA staff with whom I have worked as a close family for 17 seasons. Thank you, CCPA!

I'm honored to acknowledge Ms. Laura for writing the Foreword and for her undying dedication and role in helping spread words on how environmental toxins are causing developmental disabilities in our society.

Also, thanks to Adrianne Smith, a retired school teacher (one very honest un-song hero) who remains a loyal client, friend and unaware healer herself.

A special thanks to my family at the Healthy Living/Life Well Institute where my business currently resides.

Also, appreciation goes to Ollie Jackson, who has stood side-by-side with me as a teacher and fellow lecturer, and who has real compassion for Mother Earth and humankind.

Thank you Robin Quinn, of Quinn's Word for Word, for your wonderful editorial support and insights.

A special thanks to **Tasheka Arceneaux Sutton of the Blackvoice Graphic Design Studio for all that you've done and for all your wonderful creativity.**

Thank you James Arneson of JAAD Book Design for your artistry and great work.

Thanks also goes to my Laura Combs CCPA co-worker and friend who was the first to read my book and render positive feed-back.

A serious heart felt thank to supporters on my special projects, for without them I would not get anywhere: Dominigue Deprima, KJLH Radio - Fritz Williams, Pro-Decor - Metanasa Moralas (my sister) Producer Jammall, Inner Light Radio - Lou Austin, client and crafty genius -Carmen Buffin, The Green Machine -Myra Wallace, "Beauty Come Forth" on line magazine - Rochelle Lucas, KJLH Radio - Tamara Yapp, Real Food Real Life - I give much love and gratitude to the KJLH Front Page Family.

Consult with Author India Holloway at Her LA Office

India's Healthy Living at the *Life Well Institute*
5835 W. Washington Blvd., Culver City, CA 90230

Her services include:

Colon Hydrotherapy

This is a gentle irrigation designed to eliminate toxic waste from the large intestine. The process helps provide a favorable environment for bacteria and microflora for digestion, and it promotes a return of normal, regular bowel movements. India brings 17 years of experience to your sessions, as well as the highest level of professional training by I-ACT, the International Association for Colon Hydrotherapists.

Nutritional counseling for:

- Digestive problems
- Colon issues
- Well-being and peace of mind

India's Total Body Detox

Includes a whirlpool bath, colonic, lymphatic massage, foot detox, bouncing on a rebounder (mini-trampoline), and time in an infra-red sauna. It's a great jump-start for people who have been toxic for a long time, are on medications, or face health challenges. India's Total Body Detox helps the body clear itself of toxicity.

Iridology

India incorporates iridology into her practice, which is the scientific analysis of patterns and structures in the iris of the eye that assists in locating areas and stages of inflammation throughout the body. This analysis of the eye reveals body constitution, inherent strengths and weaknesses, health levels, and transitions that take place in a person's body according to their way of life.

Ear Candling

This natural, wholistic treatment alleviates the pain and pressure associated with sinusitis, ear aches, swimmer's ear, allergies, middle-ear infections, hearing difficulties and itching in the ear.

Detox Foot Bath

The foot bath is an all natural way to detox as your body relaxes.
To schedule an appointment with India for any of these services,

call 323-937-7300
or e-mail **indiashealthyliving@gmail.com.**

Listen to India's Weekly Radio Show
The Clean Machine

Tune in via the Internet **each Wednesday from 10 to 11 am PST** for an informative and light-hearted discussion of the health issues that can make a real difference in your life. Go to Inner Light Radio at **http://innerlightradio.com/** for health news you can use for better daily well-being.

Book India to Speak
to Your Group or Your Employees
India Holloway is also a seasoned Lecturer/Guest Speaker/ Keynote Presenter.

She lectures on health issues for women and men on a regular basis at the Life Well Institute and at other locations as a guest speaker or keynote presenter. India has appeared at the National Youth Leadership Forum on the UCLA campus, the West Angeles Church of God in Christ with the Guru of Nutrition, Dick Gregory, and KJLH's annual Women's Health Forum, as well as many other venues. A dynamic and entertaining speaker, she also presents health information to employees by invitation at businesses, such as KCET TV in Los Angeles.

To book India Holloway,
call **323-937-7300**
or e-mail **indiashealthyliving@gmail.com.**